THE NO-DIET BOOK

EAT HEALTHY AND LIVE LONGER.

GEORGE C. MIHALACHE

ISBN-10: 1983576042
ISBN-13: 978-1983576041

DEDICATION

For all my free athletes' friends, keep training! No excuses!

CONTENTS

ACKNOWLEDGMENTS

Special thanks to my parents, for keeping my curiosity alive, to my brother
who pushed me to continue writing, and to my close friends.

CHAPTER 1

THE THEORY OF HEALTHY EATING

In the old times, the food was considered a gift from the Gods, Light embedded and becoming solid, and if we think that in many cultures they were eating mostly vegetarian, this it is not far from the truth. But that was back then, and humanity went a long way in the search of progress (or not, this it is still debatable, but not right now), and today it is very important to learn about food and nutrition, in times where fast food and pre-packed, frozen meals are found everywhere, and most of us will feel nostalgic, thinking at the way our grandma use to cook from scratch, providing heartwarming meals for the whole family.

We will leave our feelings apart and connect in an intellectual way, because in this new era of information, let's face it, Knowledge is Power. The power to become much healthier, energized, ready to achieve our full potential. Here we go!

In this chapter I will try to explain how diet is linked to health. I will define the term "healthy diet", I will describe the differences in healthy diets for adults and children, I will speak about the lifestyle diseases associated with an unhealthy diet, identify sources of energy from food and tell you how much is supplied by different sources, learn to estimate your own BMR (basal metabolic rate) and PAL (physical activity level), and use this to determine energy requirements, talk about factors affecting personal energy requirements, show the relationship between energy intake, expenditure and weight gain. I will also explain why I consider that it is very important to control your salt intake.

I know, I may sound very technical, but I will put it all here, in simple words, using many examples, so you can apply it for your own benefit. I want you to wish to have a balanced and healthy diet, and that will make you to feel good, have plenty of energy and avoid unnecessary health risks. First of all, you need to know there is no One food plan that suits everybody. Each individual is unique, having slightly different nutrients requirements, depending on each one lifestyle and genetics. You will also find that age affects diet, and people of different ages need different kind and amount of food. Each person dietary requirement will change as circumstances change. For example, people who have gone through some major operations or people who get ill may require diet changes, certain illnesses or health conditions may require one to eat less or more of certain foods. For example, diabetics need to take care of their sugar and carbohydrates intake. Pregnant women need to have additional calories, vitamins and minerals to support the developing baby.

The levels or type and frequency of activity done by some person every day will result in making a diet to be healthy or unhealthy, a healthy diet for a World champion sprinter will look very different from a computer data operator who goes to gym once per week. A healthy diet need to cover all your body needs, and provide you all the nutrients required to stay healthy. What do you think about your diet? Is it healthy, almost healthy or completely unhealthy?

We will focus first on diets for children under 5, because they usually get the food their parents, or legal guardians, buy it or prepare it for them. So, the education we provide need to be directed to their families, being of paramount importance to help them to learn the good habits of eating well and balanced, so they will know how to adopt a healthy diet for their entire life. All children should have fresh food, mostly fruits, vegetables, whole grains, starchy foods (such as pasta or potatoes) and good quality protein (which can be provided by a vegetarian or normal diet. They also need plenty of fluids, from water, milk or natural juice (fizzy or sugary drinks is better to be avoided). Children caloric need is lower than an adult, but not as lower as you would think. A child between ages 1 to 3 needs on average 1200 calories per day, while a child between ages 4 to 6 should get 1600-1700 calories per day. Anyway, they should have smaller portions of food, not same size as adults. Salt should not be used in young child food, because everything that is needed is already present in other foods. Always remember that a baby kidney cannot cope with high levels of salt. Talking about this, never add processed sugar to your baby food, because if you introduce sugar in his diet too early you can condition your child to a preference for sweet foods, and potentially lead him to health issues. Fruits contain safe levels of sugars, but you should never give sugary or fizzy drink, as a baby he should drink only milk or water. Until they are 6 months old, all they need is baby milk. One healthy child should drink at least 600 ml of milk every day, until they reach 12 months. After age of one, they can safely drink cow milk. This should be full fat, as they need the fats and calories to sustain growth. Milk will provide all the nutrients needed for the first six months, but after this time the baby will grow and ask for change, meaning that they will need a more varied diet. Solid food is more difficult to digest and also contain more salt than milk. Starting solid food too early can cause stomach cramps, illness, allergies, even internal bleeding and long term damage. From 6 to 9 months, children can eat mashed and finger food like potatoes, vegetables and fruits, pieces of cheese, yogurt and pieces of toast or similar food cut into strips. At 9 months the baby should be able to eat small portions of chopped pasta, rice, beans and pulses. Probably you can try meat or fish, but I, personally, wouldn't do it. A lack of vitamin D and calcium can result in a bone disease named rickets and a lack of iron in the diet can result in anemia. Children under age of 5 should not eat too much fiber, as this can prevent them from eating other food much richer in nutrients. Some health professionals recommend a preventive dose of vitamin A and D if needed, for the ones under 5.

Children between the age of 5 and 12 will have a different nutrition, with more choice and variety than other age groups. As they are developing, they will need the same amount of healthy food as the adults, but much more vitamins and minerals to support grow. What do they need extra? We are talking about more whole grains, healthy sources of proteins and much more calcium. It is also very important for them to try a lot of different kind of foods, experiencing this will help them to find food that they like and can lead to a preference for more types of tastes. Doing this now will make it easier for them to get the right nutrients and encourage healthy eating habits later in life. My experience, when I was 18 I was always thinking that is very hard to have a vegetarian diet, as I would know only a handful of recipes. But now, after I was exposed to Chinese, Indian, Middle East, South America and many other kind of vegetarian meals, seems to be a pleasure to have so many choices, and it is also make it very easier to get the right amount of nutrients. Children at this age are still growing, not as fast as in the first five years of their life, but enough to need a complete and complex diet. They have small stomachs, but they fill and empty faster than an adult. So they need to eat every 3-4 hours, and their calories intake should be adequate. The moment will come when they will be ready to start school, then they will need to adopt a diet higher in fibre and lower in fat. Their iron intake should be closely watched, 6-7 mg at age 4-6, 8-10 mg for those aged 7-10. Salt intake for age 4 to 6, no more than 3 g a day, age 11 and more, a maximum of 6 g a day. Every parent who is cooking for a child must know that their needs vary with age.

Teenagers, what a hassle! A child gain 50% of his adult weight and 25% of his adult height during adolescence. As a result of his accelerated growth and rapid change during all this time, the nutritional and dietary requirements are also changing. The maximum recommended daily amount of iron for 11-18 years old males is 8-11 mg a day, for 11-18 years old females is 10-15 mg a day. Teenagers need to get enough iron as this nutrient is sustaining growth. Teenage girls need even more because of their particular needs. Salt for every child over age of 11, and for adults, is maximum 6 g a day (2.5 g sodium).What about calories? Oh, this is interesting, adolescents need on average 2500-2750 calories for boys and 2200 calories for girls, and best way to have it is via lean protein, low fat dairy, whole grains, fruits and vegetables. For a normal teenager to grow and maintain muscles up, he or she will need 45-55 g a day. Most adolescents easily got them from meat, fish and dairy, but vegetarians and vegans need to increase the protein intake form non animal sources like soy foods, beans, rice and nuts. Many teenagers do not get an optimum amount of calcium, leading late in life to weaker bones and osteoporosis. A parent should know that sugary foods and fizzy drinks use calcium from the bones and educate the teen to eat and drink accordingly. They need 800-1000 mg of calcium daily, and the best sources are dairy and calcium rich foods like sesame seeds or spinach. Adolescents are the group age that is the most at risk to develop eating disorders. We will talk at large about this in another chapter. Just for a short list, what are some of the important types of food they should eat: milk, cheese, yogurt, soya beans, tofu and nuts for calcium, oily fish as supplements for vitamin D (but enjoying staying outside during the day is most effective), pulses, green vegetables and cereals for iron, foods containing folate – the folic acid in natural form – as green vegetable and brown rice, for vitamin C, especially with an iron rich meal, citrus fruits, tomatoes and potatoes. What to avoid: fish (especially shark, swordfish and marlin) as these contain high levels of mercury which might affect a teenager developing nervous system, foods high in fat (saturated fat), sugar and salt should be eaten in very small amounts. Salt, no more than 6g per day, as is affecting kidneys health. For a healthy weight they need to be active and to create the habit of keeping a balanced diet, cutting down sweets, cakes, biscuits and fizzy drink, eat less fatty foods as burgers and fried food, using high quality oil for frying, regular balanced meals, based on starchy foods, wholegrain as often as possible, and many fruits and vegetables. It is more important to eat healthy and be active than to try to lose weight. If you are vegetarian or vegan, you need to include all the necessary nutrients in your diet. It is suggested to include alternative sources of protein, as milk, cheese, eggs and pulses. Also is good to get your recommended amount of minerals and vitamins.

Adults, that will be us, the majority, and what we need is a balanced diet that will provide all we need to stay fit and healthy. However, most of the adults in UK are overweight, and most probable cause is overeating (more calories than we should have daily) and lack of exercise. It is supposed to have a diet with full of fresh fruit and vegetables, proper amount of protein, starchy foods and just a bit of fat. Fat is good if is a reasonable quantity, polisaturated and unsaturated fats should have precedence to saturated fats. Saturated fat is usually found in high processed foods like cakes, biscuits and ready meals. Sugar and salt in excess can cause obesity and high blood pressure, and in some cases even cardio-vascular problems. Sugar is a good source of energy if we get it from natural products like fruits, bee honey or maple syrup, but not so good when is added to food and drinks by manufacturers. Fiber is also important for a proper digestive function, helping to prevent some lifestyle-associated diseases like heart disease. Eating our five a day portions of fruits and veggies will usually provide all our daily dose of vitamins and minerals, helping in the same time to reduce the risk of diabetes and some kind of cancers. Also, they have lot of fiber, aiding a healthy digestion.

Now I will look and compare what is needed for a healthy diet for children and for adults too. There are some differences between the optimum choice to be made daily, and I will try to point them out. A balanced diet for adults must provide all the nutrients the body needs to stay fit and healthy. A balanced diet for adults must provide all the nutrients the body needs to stay fit and healthy, but also to support growth. While adults and teenagers need a low fat diet, children under 5 will need a higher amount of fat, coming from food that also provide other nutrients, like for example full fat milk. Children should drink special formula milk until they are one year old, after that they can drink full fat milk, once they are two or more, they should gradually change it to semi-skimmed mild. Adults and teenagers should have plenty of fibre-rich food, but eating too much of them as child can prevent them to eat enough food containing the other nutrients. So, foods and drinks provide the energy we need to go about our daily lives but consuming more energy than what we need, over a longer period of time, will cause weight gain. In the UK, over 60% of adults are overweight or obese and there is concern about the number of children who are overweight. Being overweight increases the risk of developing diabetes, heart disease and some cancers in adulthood, and so maintaining a healthy weight is important for health.

The "Eat well" plate shows how foods can be classified into five groups shown as wedges of different size. These illustrate the proportions in which we should eat foods from these groups to provide a healthy diet that supplies all the nutrients our bodies need to work efficiently. You will notice that the foods in the two largest groups are all derived from plants.

Each of the groups provides a different range of essential nutrients, emphasizing the importance of a varied diet. No single food or even a single food group can provide everything we need. Also, missing out a whole food group from the main four can make it more difficult to achieve a balanced diet. Except for some people under medical supervision, no foods need to be excluded altogether. But as is explained below, some foods are best considered as treats and eaten only in small amounts or infrequently. The global population is increasing, which puts pressure on valuable resources, including food and water. In turn, food production, along with other aspects of modern living such as cars, results in greenhouse gas emissions that influence climate change. So, to ensure that there is enough food for future generations, it is important to consider the 'sustainability' of the diets we eat as well as whether or not the overall diet is healthy. By 'sustainable' we mean that the impact the production of the food has on the environment is limited. The type of diet illustrated by the "eat well" plate, which includes lots of plant-based foods, has been suggested to be relatively sustainable, especially if the fruits and vegetables consumed are those that are in season. We will always need to try to adapt our diet to the current life stage we are. The life stages are, in order: children, teenager, young man or woman, menopause, elderly, each of them having a specific approach to what we eat and drink.

Having an unhealthy diet with often result in cause some health conditions and make them worse. Obesity have been rising constantly in the last 25 years, over half of the entire UK population is overweight, with 25% clinically obese. Because of this, they got greater risk of developing problems like heart disease, diabetes, angina, and lower back or joint pain. Heart disease is one of the top causes of health problems. Bad cholesterol attaches and hardens on the inside if the tiniest blood vessel walls, which narrows them and reduce the blood flow to the heart. This can lead to ischemia, angina, or even hearth attack or strokes. Risk factors increase by age, depending on gender and family history. Some lifestyle factors can increase the odds of how likely one can develop a heart disease. Obesity can lead to 50% more chances to develop colon cancer. Smoking is another lifestyle associated with cancer. One 20 cigarettes a day smoker is 40% more likely to develop lung, throat or mouth cancer than a non-smoker. Yearly, more than 250.000 people are diagnosed with cancer. Most common ones are breast, lung, bowel or prostate. Diabetes, if it is not managed successfully, can lead to blindness, kidney failure, foot ulceration, nerve damage and even heart problems. One with diabetes cannot use glucose properly, but this illness can be managed with medication and diet. Type 2 diabetes (insulin dependent) is linked with obesity, so eating healthy and exercising can significantly reduce the risk of Type 2. Tooth decay is very common nowadays, half of UK population suffers from some kind of tooth decay, and the main cause being the acids coming from fermented sugar and starches, acid that is breaking down the tooth. Young children are very vulnerable to tooth decay, as their enamel is still developing. Adults will suffer from tooth decay because enamel has been worn down.

But coming back to obesity – defined as a term used to describe somebody who is very overweight, with a lot of body fat. It's a common problem, estimated to affect around one in every four adults and around one in every five children aged 10 to 11 in the UK. How we define someone as being obese? Well, there are many ways in which a person's health in relation to their weight can be classified, but the most widely used method is body mass index (BMI). BMI is a measure of whether you're a healthy weight for your height. You can use the BMI healthy weight calculator to work out your score. For most adults:
-a BMI of 25 to 29.9 means you are considered overweight
-a BMI of 30 to 39.9 means you are considered obese
-a BMI of 40 or above means you are considered severely obese

BMI is not used to definitively diagnose obesity – as people who are very muscular sometimes have a high BMI, without excess fat – but for most people, it can be a useful indication of whether they may be overweight. A better measure of excess fat is waist circumference, and can be used as an additional measure in people who are overweight (with a BMI of 25 to 29.9) or moderately obese (with a BMI of 30 to 34.9). Generally, men with a waist circumference of 94 cm or more and women with a waist circumference of 80 cm or more are more likely to develop obesity-related health problems. Obesity is generally caused by consuming more calories – particularly those in fatty and sugary foods – than you burn off through physical activity. The excess energy is then stored by the body as fat. Obesity is an increasingly common problem, because many modern lifestyles often promote eating excessive amounts of cheap, high-calorie food and spending a lot of time sitting at desks, on sofas or in cars. There are also some underlying health conditions that can occasionally contribute to weight gain, such as an underactive thyroid gland (hypothyroidism), although conditions such as this don't usually cause weight problems if they are effectively controlled with medication. The best way to treat obesity is to eat a healthy, reduced-calorie diet and to exercise regularly.

To do this you should:
-eat a balanced, calorie-controlled diet as recommended by your GP or weight loss management health professional (such as a dietician).
-join a local weight loss group.
-take up activities such as fast walking, jogging, swimming or tennis for 150-300 minutes a week.
-eat slowly and avoid situations where you know you could be tempted to overeat.

You may also benefit from psychological support from a trained healthcare professional, to help change the way you think about food and eating. In rare cases, weight loss surgery may be recommended.

Next point on the list is energy provided by what we eat. Our body uses the nutrients from the food as energy. Energy is measured in calories. One calorie is the amount of energy needed to raise the temperature of 1 g of water with 1° C. A calorie is the basic unit to measure energy that we use to walk, talk, breathe, sleep or run. All of our activities use energy, burning calories. Our food contains calories, coming from carbohydrates, fats or proteins. These nutrients are measured in grams, each gram defined by a number of calories. Our body needs a defined amount of calories in order to work properly. Everything we do, every action or non-action, like breathing or sleeping, all of them burn calories. The rate that these calories are consumed is called Basal Metabolic Rate (BMR). The relation between calories and weight is this, for every 3500 calories you eat in excess of your daily activities, you will get one lb. of body fat, every 3500 calories we use on top of our daily activities, we lose 1 lb. in body fat. As for nutrients, for every gram of it, we got 4 calories for carbohydrates and proteins, and 9 calories for fats. The Basal Metabolic Rate (BMR), if we define it, is the rate at which a person uses energy to maintain the basic functions of the body (keeping warm, heart activity and breathing included). Not all of us have the same BMR. Every person use on average 1.1 calories every minute just to breathe, heart beat and stay warm. A person's BMR is usually about ¾ of one's energy needs. But toddlers and young children will have a high BMR due to their rapid growth and development. If you got more muscle mass, you will have a higher BMR as it takes more energy to maintain muscles. More muscles, more energy you use. As you get old, your BMR will decrease for the same reason, muscle mass decreasing with age.

Case study 001: John and Beatrice
In order to calculate their BMR, we will need age, height and weight.
John aged 36, 6' tall, 169 lbs. Beatrice aged 33, 5'8" tall, 141 lbs.

The formula we need to use is:
Male BMR = 66+(6.23 x weight in pounds)+(12.7 x height in inches)-(6.8 x age in years)
Female BMR = 655+(4.35 x weight in pounds)+(4.7 x height in inches)-(4.7 x age in years)

After we calculate their BMR the result is: John
66+(6.23 x 169)+(12.7 x 72)-(6.8 x 36)=
66+1052.87+914.4-244.8=
1788.47 kcal
Beatrice
655+(4.35 x 141)+(4.7 x 68)-(4.7 x 33)=
655+613.35+319.6-155.1=
1440.85 kcal

It is very important to remember that BMR is affected by one's physical activity levels (PAL). Try now to calculate your own basal metabolic rate (BMR). Do it right here, right now.

....

....

....

Is it too hard? You can use this link:
www.bmi-calculator.net/bmr-calculator/ or you can make your own excel file to do this.

Physical activity levels

Everything you do is burning calories. Most of the calories are used for basics, the other ones are burned through exercises and other activities. You will burn calories even after an activity has stopped. By combining basal requirements with needs based on physical activity levels, you can calculate your total energy requirement. The more activity a person does, the more energy is burned. The way to calculate your total energy requirement is:

Total Energy Needed = BMR x PAL

One's PAL is determined by the things a person does in a 24 hours period. It can also be estimated when you know the activities you perform that day. Each activity is connected to a particular level of activity.

Level 1: Sedentary
This level of activity is when you do little or no exercise. PAL factor is 1.2.
Level 2: Light exercise
This level of activity is described by you doing frequent walking in a job/daily activity or 60 minutes of intense activity in one week. PAL factor is 1.375.
Level 3: Moderate exercise
This level of activity could include a job that is quite physical through the day or intense physical activity of 30-60 minutes three – four times a week. PAL factor is 1.55.
Level 4: Very active
Thus level of activity could be a highly physical job such as brick laying or farming or intense exercise for 60 minutes five to seven days a week. PAL factor is 1.725.
Level 5: Extreme
This level of activity includes full time training for a sporting event, usually reached only by elite athletes. PAL factor is 1.9.

Case study
John and Beatrice

John and Beatrice will work out their physical activity levels. John is a very active person with a PAL factor of 1.725. However Beatrice has a very sedentary life, so his PAL factor is 1.2. Now that John and Beatrice have calculated their BMR and PAL, they can work out their energy requirements using Harris Benedict formula:
Energy requirement = BMR x PAL

John and Beatrice use this to work out the number:

	BMR	PAL factor	Energy requirement
John	1788.47	1.725	3085.11
Beatrice	1440.85	1.2	1729.02

Now John and Beatrice found their daily energy requirements and they can use it to plan a healthy balanced diet, to make sure they do not gain or lose too much weight.

Make sure that you are doing this at least every 6 months, to estimate your own energy requirements. In the last 40 years we slowly went form a very active life to one where we are not doing much physical activity. In the past, many jobs were physically demanding, construction, agriculture, you name it, all of them requiring a large amount of physical effort. Now most of the jobs are desk based (more than 53%), and even on the non-desk based jobs, more than 90% admit that they sit down most of the time.

It is recommended to do at least 150 minutes of moderate intensity aerobic activity every week, adding muscle strengthening activities on two or more days. It can be spread across the week, such as 30 minutes a day over 5 days. But what is moderate intensity aerobic activity you would ask? Activities classed as moderately intense are: golf, tennis, skateboarding, swimming or volleyball. Another alternative could be 75 minutes of vigorous intensity aerobic activity and muscle strengthening activities two or more days. Vigorous intensity aerobic activities examples are: aerobics, football (not as keeper), basketball, hockey or running. But is important to do a mix of moderate/vigorous aerobics and muscle strengthening exercises (anything that helps to build muscle as press ups, sit ups, weight lifting, yoga or something similar). If you understand how the different activity levels can help you understand your own energy requirements, you will be able to remain fit and healthy. This is more important for busy mums, families, young people, office workers, older adults and disabled people.

You can walk more, use 10 minutes sessions few times a day, start running or cycle, use stairs instead of lift, stand when talk on the phone or use your imagination to avoid more than 1 hour sitting. Once you can calculate your total energy requirements you are in a position to maintain your own weight. If you are taking on more energy that you are using, the extra calories will be converted in fat, in order to lose weight you need to use more energy than you consume. Look at the food you are eating and find ways to decrease the amount of calories that you consume. You can cut out certain foods or use low calorie alternatives. You can increase your activity, taking up exercise or sport. Use these two methods together, and you will achieve results much faster. Increasing your energy requirements and reducing your calorie intake is the key to the perfect weight.

Case study - Alexander

Alexander is 40 lbs. overweight. His PAL is around 1.5. His BMR is 2200 calories per day and his total energy requirement is 3300 calories. However, he eats about 4000 calories every day. He is continuing to put on weight. Alexander wants to lose weight. He starts by increasing his exercise regime so that his PAL is 1.8.

This means his energy requirement becomes:

2200 x 1.8 = 3960 calories

We just talk about using both methods, reducing calorie intake and increasing physical activity, as the best strategy. If Alexander keeps on eating the same amount but increases his activity level, he will more or less stop putting on weight. However, if he decided to eat 10% (400 calories per day) less he would lose about 1 lb. every 9 days. In a year this will be close to his target weight!

Salt intake and blood pressure

Salt is present in most of the foods, and same like sugar, many are not aware of this. When you add more salt for taste, this can result in an increase of daily recommended amount. If a person eats too much salt, it can lead to raised blood pressure. This may increase the likelihood of someone suffering from heart disease and strokes. If a person eats a safe amount of salt then the risk of these problems developing is minimized. A special warning about children! When they are very young, their kidneys can find it difficult to deal with more than 1 g of salt per day. Giving children too much salty food can mean that they develop a taste for it and are more likely to eat too much salt when they are adults. Most of the pre-packed and processed meals already contain salt, so monitoring will prove to be difficult. Is not always easy to find out, some will have a higher salt content, others will vary according to manufacturer or brand. What you need to know? Almost always high in salt content: bacon, cheese, gravy granules, ham, pickled, prawns, salami, and salted nuts. Following foods can be high in salt content: breakfast cereals, crisps, crumpets, bagels, pasta sauces, ketchup, mayo, sausages, ready meals, pizza.

How much is recommended?

Under 9 months – none
9-12 months – 1 g
1-3 year   – 2 g
4-6 year   – 3 g
7-10 year   – 5 g
11+ years   – 6 g

Components of a healthy diet

Short story: I will just point it out what are they, main nutritional benefits, how much we should have each day, what are they and add some interesting informations.

1. Fruit and vegetables: they contain notable quantities of vitamins, minerals and fibre. We should eat 33% of our daily meals or 5 portions equivalent. Not only fresh, frozen and tinned are also included. Note: Potatoes are a carbohydrate, not a vegetable.

2. Protein-rich products: contain protein, vitamins and minerals, we should have a percentage of 15% daily or 2-3 portions equivalent.

3. Fatty or sugary foods: the main nutritional benefit is that they are providing energy, we should have no more than 4% daily, meaning one portion or less. Include sweets, cakes, and biscuits

4. Milk and dairy: the main benefit is that can provide protein and calcium, we should eat approx. 15% or 2-3 portions. Most useful are yogurt, cheese and milk.

5. Carbohydrates: the main nutritional benefit is that can provide energy, fibre, vitamins and minerals. The average proportion is 33% or a third of our diet. We include here bread, cereals, potatoes, pasta, beans and lentils.

The reason we need a diet drawn from all of the groups is that they all deliver different, but vital, nutritional benefits to our bodies. Fruit and vegetables are one of our main sources of vitamins and minerals, which the body needs to perform a variety of functions well. For instance, vitamin A helps to strengthen our immune system, B vitamins help us process energy from food, vitamin D helps us maintain healthy teeth and bones, and vitamin C helps to keep cells and tissues healthy. The steamed carrots and broccoli, pictured above, will maintain a higher proportion of vitamins than boiled or fried vegetables. Fruit and vegetables (eaten with the skin on) also contain high amounts of fibre which help to maintain a healthy gut and digestive system. Starchy foods, also known as carbohydrates, are where we get most of our energy from. Our bodies convert these foods into glucose which is used as energy either immediately or stored for later use. Carbohydrates also contain fibre (especially wholegrain), and iron which we need to make red blood cells to carry oxygen around the body. Meat fish, eggs and pulses provide us with significant amounts of protein which is essentially a building block of the body. Everything from our hair, muscles, nerves, skin and nails needs protein to build and repair itself. The grilled mackerel, pictured, is an excellent source. Also high in protein are dairy products, and they are also great providers of calcium. The most common mineral in the body, calcium is needed for functions including helping blood to clot, and to build bones and teeth. Fortunately, the fatty and sugary group, the foods that we find the most irresistible, also have a role to play, in moderation. Fat transports the fat-soluble vitamins A, D, E and K around the body. It also cushions and protects the internal organs. Sugar is another food that gives us energy, whether it's the naturally occurring fructose sugars in fruit or sucrose in table sugar. But probably other healthy sources of energy are better to be preferred, as white sugar is known to deplete out body of some vitamins and minerals in the process of their assimilation.

Try to base meals on starchy carbohydrates such as bread, pasta or potatoes. Include a range of different fruit and vegetables in your diet and try to have at least one to two portions with every meal. Including a moderate serving of protein-containing food is also important. Then choose adequate calcium sources, aiming for three portions of low-fat dairy or dairy alternatives daily. Whilst a small amount of sugary foods each day is acceptable, eating sugar too frequently may increase risk of tooth decay. Weight gain may also occur if sugar in the diet provides more energy than we are using up. And many dieticians agree there's no such thing as a 'superfood'. The overall balance of the diet is what really matters, and guides such as the Eatwell Plate can be helpful. No single food will provide all the nutrients we really need. And neither can one meal - so the plate of food above might be one healthy option, but a good diet should include a wide range of foods from each of the different food groups. Fluids are also vital to help our bodies perform their functions effectively, and the best fluid of all is water. Two-thirds of a healthy human body is actually made up of water. It's necessary to help our blood carry nutrients and waste around the body and to help the chemical reactions that occur in our cells.

What are the most recommended tips for eating well? I will tell you some of them. You know that starchy foods include bread, pasta, beans, peas and lentils. But better remember that wholegrain, or wholemeal varieties contain more vitamins and minerals than white sources. Eat lots of fruit and vegetables. There is scientific evidence that people who do this are at lower risk of heart disease, strokes and even cancers. For the pescetarians, fish is an important source of protein, and contains many vitamins and minerals. It's also rich in omega-3 fatty acids. People can choose from fresh, frozen or canned. However, some canned and smoked fish can be high in salt. Eating too much sugar can lead to weight gain. Excess weight gain can lead to obesity and increased risks of diseases including Type 2 diabetes, heart disease and some cancers. Sugar is found naturally in lots of foods, but it is also often added to foods like fizzy drinks, cakes, biscuits, chocolate, pastries etc. It is better to exchange white sugar with brown one, honey or maple syrup. Eating too much fat can lead to weight gain. Excess weight gain can lead to obesity and increased risks of diseases including Type 2 diabetes, heart disease and some cancers. There are two main kinds of fat, but it is saturated fat that people should cut down on. Saturated fat is found in food like pies, processed meat, cheese, cake and biscuits. It can raise your blood cholesterol and increase the risk of heart disease. Unsaturated fat can help to lower cholesterol and provide people with essential fatty acids needed to stay healthy. Sources of unsaturated fats include oily fish, nuts and seeds, avocados, olive oils and vegetable oils. Guidelines recommend that you eat no more than 6 g of salt each day. You should avoid adding salt to your food where possible, as ¾ of the salt we need is already in the food we buy. Getting enough exercise is an important way of keeping your weight at a healthy level. It can also help to reduce the risk of some diseases. You'll learn more about this in the following pages. It's important that women drink about 1.6 litres of water a day and men drink about 2 liters of water a day. A healthy breakfast is an important part of a balanced diet. Some research shows that eating a balanced breakfast can actually help you to control your weight!

Case study - Christopher Smith

Chris has decided that he wants to make a change to his lifestyle. He is obese, drinks at least thirty pints of beer a week, has takeaway food 5 or 6 times a week and smokes 15 cigarettes a day – this makes him feel tired, lethargic and generally unhealthy. Chris visited his doctor to ask for some advice on changing his lifestyle. He knows that his current lifestyle could make him ill and even shorten his life. The doctor outlined some changes that could be made, but understood that Chris would need to change gradually as a very large sudden change in lifestyle may be difficult to keep up in the long term. What changes does Chris make? He learn about habit change and used opposite healthy habits to be reinforced as he decreased the wrong ones in frequency. First he stopped smoking, then he start to cook healthy nutritious meals at home, while he started to drink less. Through time Chris and the doctor sought to gradually improve Chris's lifestyle so that his health would keep improving. After six months, Chris had lost 5 stones and had quit smoking; he drank far less alcohol and felt like a much healthier person.

The 5 a day initiative encourages people in the UK to eat a minimum of 5 portions of fruit and vegetables every day. Many people don't eat enough fruit and vegetables, but they are an essential part of a healthy diet. Almost all fruit and vegetables count towards your 5 a day. They don't have to be fresh to count as a portion, and can be included as part of a meal. Each adult portion should be roughly 80 g. Click the slider to learn more about your 5 a day.
- Fruit and vegetables - These can be fresh, frozen or tinned. Tinned fruit / vegetables should be in natural juice or water. Fruit and veg can be cooked in soups, stews or pasta dishes.
- Dried fruit - All dried fruit counts towards your 5 a day. This could include things like currents, dates and raisins.
- Fruit juice - Juice only ever counts as one portion a day, even if you drink more than one glass of it! This is because juice contains less fibre than whole fruits and vegetables.
- Smoothies - A smoothie containing all of the edible pulped fruit and/or vegetables can count as a maximum of two portions per day.
- Beans and pulses - this only count as one portion a day, no matter how many you eat. They contain fewer nutrients than other fruits and vegetables.
- Pre-packaged meals - These may be high in sugar, salt and fat. It helps to check food labels when eating some of your 5 a day in this way.
- Root vegetables - Potatoes don't count as one of your five a day, and neither do yams, cassava or plantain. This is because they are starchy foods, which are rich in energy and fibre. However, other root vegetables such as sweet potato, parsnips and turnips do count!

And just in case you struggle with your 5-a-day, here are some ideas for you:

1. A lamb and vegetable kebab - Up to 2 portions. Kebabs are a super barbecue option - you can add mushrooms, peppers and onions. Don't forget corn cobs can be finished on the barbecue too. Add a bowl of salad and you've chalked up an extra portion.

2. Baked beans on toast - Better-than-baked beans add up for 1 portion. Pulses (lentils or beans) of any type count as one portion. Top with a sliced tomato for a tasty two-portion snack.

3. Avocado & chili salad - An avocado, prosciutto and tomato salad will add up to 3 portions. Half an avocado counts as one portion. Add two large tomatoes and a handful of salad leaves and you're three portions ahead!

4. Seven cup muesli - Cereal topped with a banana count as 1 portion. A simple way to get an extra portion a day: slice a banana on top of that morning cereal.

5. Apricots - A mini packet of raisins counts as 1 portion. Around ½ to 1 tablespoon of currants, raisins or two dried apricots or prunes is the equivalent of one portion.

6. Breakfast smoothie - A smoothie (with whole fruits is best) counts as up to 2 portions. A smoothie counts as at least one portion - often two or more. But how can you tell? Go for those with lots of information on the label. Smoothies made from whole fruits are best, as they contain fibre.

7. Blueberry milkshakes - A home-made blueberry milkshake will provide 2 portions. Home-made shakes help pile up the portions. However, takeaway shakes made without real fruit don't count. As 80 g of blueberries equals one portion, it should be easy to make a two-portion shake. The vegetables have to add up to 80 g to count as a portion, so you'll need one large tomato and a generous helping of cucumber to make up the weight.

8. Chicken stir fry - Chicken and vegetable stir fry will provide 2-3 portions It's easy to get two or even three portions of vegetables into a stir fry, so go for a wide and colorful selection - red and green peppers, onion, broccoli, beansprouts, sweet potatoes and so on.

9. Gazpacho - New Covent Garden Soup ads up to 2-3 portions. It varies between flavors, but their Fresh Gazpacho contains 256 g of tomatoes, 74 g of cucumber and 74 g of red pepper - half a carton is a two to three-portion lunch or supper.

10. Cherries - Two handfuls of cherries or grapes made 1 portion. Make a change from an apple a day: always make the most of whatever fresh fruit is in season.

11. Strawberries in lime syrup - A small punnet of strawberries will provide 1 portion. Wimbledon wouldn't be Wimbledon without strawberries. Try topping with crème fraiche or Greek yogurt.

12. Summer sandwiches - A cheese, tomato and cucumber sandwich will give you 1 portion. The vegetables have to add up to 80 g to count as a

portion so you'll need one large tomato and a generous helping of cucumber to make up the weight.

Variety and the hidden health impact

There are many advantages to eating a wide variety of foods. A narrower range can be unhealthy, less enjoyable and more expensive. If people want to stay healthy, they need to meet a variety of nutritional needs. These needs can't be met by just one food! People should eat a variety of different foods to make sure they get everything they need. For example, a person who only ate brown rice and apples would be missing out on many essential nutrients. This lack of variety would lead to an unhealthy diet. When there is little variation in meals, a person may be more likely to eat unhealthily. Eating a wide variety of healthy foods will help a person eat healthily. By liking a range of different foods, people are in an easier position to choose healthy options rather than unhealthy ones. People who eat a limited range of foods may struggle with their diet if the food they eat becomes unavailable or is in short supply. They may have difficulty getting all the nutrients they need. If a person likes a variety of foods, they have more choice over what to eat. Someone who eats a wide variety of foods has a better chance of finding the nutrition they need in the food available.

So far you have looked at different foods and how they link to health and diet. Now you will learn more about the nutrients in these foods, and how they contribute to a healthy body. There are different classes of nutrients. They are all very important and all have different purposes. Different people need different amounts of nutrients at different development stages in their lives. It's also important to stay hydrated. Water plays a key part in hydration.

The six classes of nutrients are:

Fruit and vegetables – main nutritional benefits are in providing vitamins, minerals and fiber. We should have them as 33% of our diet or 5 portions. Fresh is preferred, but you can also include frozen or tinned.

Protein – main nutritional benefits are in providing protein, vitamins and minerals. We should have them as 15% of our diet or 2-3 portions.

Fatty or sugary foods – provide energy. We should have them as 4% of our diet or 1 portion or less. These include sweets, cakes, and biscuits.

Milk and dairy – main nutritional benefits are in providing protein and calcium. We should have them as 15% of our diet or 2-3 portions. These include yogurt, cheese and milk.

Carbohydrates - main nutritional benefits are in providing energy, fiber, vitamins and minerals. We should have them as 33% of our diet. These include bread, cereal, potatoes, pasta, beans, and lentils.

Many people have a chaotic choice when we talk about our daily diet. We often eat and drink too many calories, too much fat, sugar and salt, not enough fruit, vegetables and fibre. What we need to do? In theory it is very easy:

- plenty of fruit and vegetables,
- plenty of starchy foods as rice, potatoes and pasta,
- eggs, beans and other non-dairy sources of protein,
- milk and dairy products, but not every day,
- small amount of foods that are high in fat and/or sugar or none at all.

There are many sources of information offering advice and tips on healthy eating, but it is best to stick to official sources of information, such as NHS website. The Food Standards Agency is a Government body for food and nutrition.

Advice for a better diet, related to the six classes of nutrients:
- wholegrain or wholemeal varieties contains more vitamins and minerals than their white equivalents;
- if you eat more vegetables and fruit, you are at lower risk of heart disease, strokes and cancer;
- for ones who are not having a vegetarian diet, fish is an important source or omega 3 fatty acids, but if it is canned or smoked can be very high in salt;
- if you eat too much sugar you can easily gain weight. Also you increase the risk of becoming obese or getting ill (type 2 diabetes, heart disease, cancer);
- if you eat too much fat you can get excess weight, increasing the risks of getting ill, in the same way as for excess sugar);
- unsatured fat is better than saturated, as you lower cholesterol and get more essential fatty acids, from sources as nuts, seeds, avocado, olive and vegetable oils;
- do not eat more than 6 g of salt daily, remember that ¾ of the salt we need we get it from the food we buy.
- being active and keeping a normal weight is useful in decreasing the risk of some diseases, we will talk about this later on;
- drinking enough water is very important, as our efficiency decrease even when we lose 5% of the bodily water;
- breakfast is important in controlling our weight, eating before 6 PM is preferred to a late dinner.

Eating a wide variety of foods is important, as a narrower range can be unhealthy, less enjoyable and much more expensive. Your needs cannot be met by just one food, the lack of variety can lead to an unhealthy diet. By eating a variety of different foods, you will be able to enjoy a wide variety of texture, flavors and combinations. Having a healthy lifestyle must be something enjoyable and appealing. When you eat a limited range of foods, you may struggle with your diet if the food you it become unavailable. If you like a variety of foods, you have a better chance of finding the nutrition you need in the food that it is available.

Nutrient classes

There are different classes of nutrients, all of them very important because they have different purposes. People need different amounts of nutrients at different development stages in their lives. Added to this, water it is also very important, playing a key part in staying hydrated.

There are six classes of nutrients. A nutrient is a chemical substance that provides nourishment to the body. They are essential for growth, development and maintain the health. The nutrients classes are carbohydrates, fats, proteins, vitamins, minerals and water. Let's explain each of them in few words.

Carbohydrates are needed when you use up energy. Your brain and body can get energy much quicker from carbohydrates than from proteins and fats. There are two main kinds of them: starches and sugars. Starches are sometimes called complex carbohydrates and are healthier than sugars. One important complex carbohydrate is fibre, which helps all the food to pass through body and has a role in digestion. Sugars can be found naturally (bee honey) or added to some foods. Foods rich in starches are pasta, bread, rice, oats, potatoes and pulses. Foods rich in sugars are fruits, vegetables or ones with added sugar as cakes and biscuits.

Fats are of two different kinds: saturated and unsaturated. Eating too much of the wrong kind of fats can lead to being overweight and to obesity. People should have a low fat diet, but to provide the necessary essential fatty acids body need to function. There are many researches that find strong links between eating saturated fats and heart disease. Saturated fats can be found in dairy products, biscuits, cakes, burgers, pies. Unsaturated fats can be found in butter, ghee, vegetable oils, and fish like tuna or sardines.

Proteins help with growth and maintain healthy bones, blood, muscles and skin. The correct daily amount of protein is very important, especially if you want to develop physically as a teenager. When you do not eat enough carbohydrates, the body can convert proteins into energy. But if you eat too much protein and not burn enough energy, the protein will be converted in fat. Proteins can be broken down into 23 amino-acids. Most of them are produced by our body, but 8 of them must come from diet. Important sources of protein are eggs, nuts, lentils, or if you are not vegetarian, fish, lean red meat, white meat.

Vitamins are important in keeping us healthy, helping our immune system or regulate the release of minerals like calcium. Our own bodies cannot synthetize vitamins, so we need to obtain them from food. Fruits, vegetables, nuts and cereals are rich in the vitamins we need every day. When we do not get enough vitamins we develop a vitamin deficiency. This can have a direct impact on bone development, tissue growth, immune system or organ optimal function. Did you know that green vegetables are a great source of vitamin B, responsible to change the nutrients from food into energy? Or that the oranges are a great source of vitamin C, that helps to fight infection and to release energy from fats?

Minerals are usually found in cereals, dairy, vegetables, fruits and nuts. They are helping us to build strong bones and teeth, controlling bodily fluids, turning our meal into energy. The two most important minerals are iron, helping with the flow of oxygen through the body, and calcium, related to strong bones and teeth. Vegetables like broccoli are rich in iron, milk and cheese have plenty of calcium, potassium, found in bananas, potatoes and tomatoes, keeps blood pressure down. Fruits and vegetables are the most common source of minerals, so if you do not eat them every day, more likely you will not get the minerals you need.

Water is the most ignored nutrient. We are, by weight, about 66% water. There is strong evidence to link dehydration to increased chance to have asthma, high blood pressure, ulcers, joint problems and high cholesterol. Poor hydration can lead to joint aches and pain, having a negative impact on our physical activity. The function of the brain (which is 85% water) and of the central nervous system is negatively affected by dehydration. It is also a known negative impact on the energy and nutrients absorption by the body. Dehydration also affects body's ability to maintain a safe temperature, risking overheating.

How do you think you can increase your fluid intake to a decent level?

-

-

-

Hydration and exercise

It is recommended to drink about 500 ml of fluids in the two hours before training, also it is important to drink early and often during exercise, so you can replace the fluids lost through sweat. After exercise it is suggested that you need to continue to replace the fluids lost due to sweat, and to combat the after-burn effect. During and after exercise that last longer than one hour, you need to replace the lost electrolytes also. Ideally is to have a drink containing electrolytes and carbohydrates. Green vegetables such as cucumber, celery or spinach have water content above 90%, so they are a great source of water.

You will need a different proportion of carbohydrates, fats and proteins, related to your personal activity level. A weightlifter has different needs than a marathon runner. Children, teenagers and adults should have by default a diet that is low in fat. The levels of activity and variations in this through the day are affecting how much of each nutrient you need. If you are ill, recovering from an injury or pregnant, then you will need different nutrients. Age is a factor too in the daily dietary requirement. If you want to lose or to gain weight, or you want to build muscle, you will need to change and adapt your dietary requirements.

Case study

Anna is trying to find out the amount of calories she and her friend should be getting from proteins. Anna found that, as a result of her lifestyle, 15% of her total calories intake should be from protein. Her friend Mario is a footballer, she works out that 25% of his calories should come from protein. Mario's brother is a professional wrestler. His trainer told him that 32 of his calories should come from proteins, because the physical demands on his body are much higher that Anna or Mario.

If you understand your need and know how to provide with the correct nutrition, you will achieve a better health and wellbeing. Are there any changes that you would make for your own lifestyle in your consumption of nutrients? Explain why you want to make/to not make any changes.

-

-

-

Case study

Susan and Victor are flat mates at university. Susan is a competitive athlete, Victor is more of a couch potato. As part of his P.A. assignment, Susan will compare her water intake with Victor.

Victor water intake:

He is not eating many water rich foods. He drinks 2-3 milky coffee a day. On occasions he will drink a small glass of water. If he goes out he will drink shots. As it is the cold season, he mostly stays in the flat with the heating on high.

Victor was consuming around 1 liter per day and he was poorly hydrated, needing to consume more liquids.

Susan water intake:

She plays competitive volleyball three times a week and trains twice a week. She will often run a 4-6 mile run at least once a week. She eats a water rich food diet. She drinks 4 x 300 ml glasses of water on the day without training. She drinks about 250-500 ml, 2-3 hours before exercise and 250 ml every 15 minutes during exercise. Weighs herself before and after exercise and replace the fluids lost.

On non-training day Susan got the amount of water she needed. On a training day Susan had a water intake of 4-5 litres depending on the intensity of training or sports activity. She was replacing the fluids she lost during exercise.

Principles of healthy food preparation

It is well known that when we are asked to choose between a balanced meal with average taste and a very tasty meal with limited nutritional value, most people would decide to have the second choice. The reason is that good tasting food gives us instant pleasure, while to see any benefits from balanced nutrients it takes a while. The good news is that it is possible to enjoy a balanced nutritional meal, if you plan accordingly.

Case study

Anita often chooses tasty, unhealthy foods over nutritionally balanced meals. She was always thinking that healthy food lack taste and because of that she never tried and enjoys it. After years of having this kind of diet, Anita begins to feel tired and her skin does not look as clear.

Her friends are encouraging her to eat more healthy, and although she does not like boiled vegetables, she prefer them as part of a meal, as a curry or a stir-fry. Even though Anita doesn't enjoy fruits, she really likes smoothies. By understanding her own preferences, she has been able to improve her diet and feel healthier on long term.

Make some notes about what you like and dislike. Could any of your preferences are for pleasure instead of nutrition? The ideal is to have your meals both nutritious and tasty. Here are some tips to inspire you. A simple way to make your own meals healthier is to use the substitution and reduction method. This involves substituting some of you key ingredients with others that are lower in fat, salt or sugar. You can use low fat yogurt or crème fraiche instead of cream. You can use brown rice instead of white one, you can use whole-wheat varieties of bread and pasta instead of white ones. Use less cheese when making pizza. Use less sugar or have maple or agave syrup instead when doing cakes and biscuits.

Case study

Daniel is 44 and wants to lose weight. He knows that he need a healthy diet and thinks that if he will build some good habits, he will reach his target faster. An important part of the achieving this goal is to substitute unhealthy food with better and healthier options. Daniel also looks to see whether he should stop eat certain food and drink alcohol altogether.

Look at Daniel's meals before and after he changed his diet.

Breakfast before changes:
Wholegrain toast with butter
Baked beans
Tomato
Glass of milk

Breakfast after changes:
Wholegrain toast with low-fat spread cheese
Baked beans
Tomato
Glass of tea

Morning break before changes:
2 Hobnobs
Bag of crisps
Coffee with milk

Morning break after changes:
Apple
Coffee with milk

Lunch before changes:
Roast beef sandwich with wholegrain bread, cheese and butter
One can of Coke

Lunch after changes:
Roast beef sandwich with wholegrain bread, low-fat spread cheese and
mixed salad
Herbal tea

Afternoon break before changes:
Bag of crisps
Chocolate bar
Coffee with milk

Afternoon break after changes:
Unsalted nuts and seeds
Coffee with milk

Evening meal before changes:
Fish in butter

French fries
Baked beans
Two cans of lager

Evening meal after changes:
Baked fish
Baked potato
Peas
Carrots
Broccoli

Evening snack before changes:
Slice of cake

Evening snack after changes:
Fruit salad with reduced fat yogurt

Daniel makes some changes in order to improve his diet. The methods he used are:

-Substitution – using low-fat spread cheese instead of butter and tea instead of milk or Coke.

-Removal – crisps, chocolate bars, lager, Coke and cake all have been removed.

-Different cooking styles – the introduction of the baked fish and potato instead of fried fish and fried chips cuts Daniel's calories from 480 to 310 and also cuts his fats intake from 24 g to 4 g. You will learn about different cooking methods in the next pages.

The result is good, the new diet removed 1400-1450 calories and approx. 26 grams of fat from Daniel's diet. He will also get more minerals and vitamins from his increased fruit and vegetable intake. Substitution and reduction methods can have a significant impact on long-term health, while allowing us to keep a similar diet.

***

There are a number of different ways of cooking and preparing our foods. Some of them are healthier than others. Let's see how we prepare the five different food groups.

Vegetables – boiling vegetables in water is not the healthiest way to cook them, as many of us would think. Steaming or stir-frying your vegetables can help them to retain more nutrients. If you need to boil them, using a smaller amount of water can help. The water used to cook vegetables can be reused for healthy stocks or gravy.

Fruits – some people do not like to eat fruits. Anyway, making them part of a fruit salad or dessert or blending those into smoothies can make them more enjoyable.

Starchy foods – when you boil potatoes, using less water can help them to retain more nutrients. You can also use aromatic herbs instead of butter or sauces to ad flavors to baked potatoes or rice. Making your own pasta sauces instead of buying it is another way to make starchy food healthier, by minimizing the amount of cream you are eating.

Meat, fish and pulses – If you need to eat meat, try to use lean cuts and remove the skin from meats like chicken, turkey or duck, in order to make it less fatty. Beans and lentils can be used to add texture and flavor to meat dishes. Choosing oily fish once a week to provide omega 3-6-9 fatty acids can be an alternative to heavy meats like pork, lamb or beef.

Daily – using low fat dairy options is a good way to lower your cholesterol. Using skimmed milk, low fat cheese and plain yogurt or crème fraiche instead of cream are good ways to decrease the fat in your diet. Yogurt instead of ice cream is a good choice also!

Fats and sugars – it is important to minimize your fat and sugar intake. Choosing unsaturated fats over saturated fats and substituting sugar with honey or maple syrup it is also a great way to do this. Remember to always check the food labels, as many processed foods have high fat and sugar content.

Salt – it is very important also to check food labels for the salt intake. You can also reduce the salt from your diet if you use herbs and spices to add flavor to your food instead of salt. Choosing crunchy vegetables as a snack instead of crisps and drinking enough water to be properly hydrated through the day can help to reduce your salt intake.

Task: Think about few ways to make your diet healthier without giving up the pleasure you get from eating your favorite meals.

———

———

———

***

Ways of cooking and preparing the food

Baking – the food is inside the oven. This method is used to make bread and cakes, as well as to cook poultry, meat and veggies.

Barbecue – the food is cooked on a rack above hot coals. Little or no fat is used and the meal has a nice smoked flavor.

Boiling – this involve placing the food in boiling water for a set period of time.

Braising – food is cooked in a small amount of water in an open or covered pan. The cooking liquid keeps the food moist.

Casserole – the food is placed in a large amount of liquid (water, stock or wine for example) and it is heated gently over an extended period of time.

Deep frying – food is placed in high temperature fats and oils.

Grilling – food is placed underneath a heat source.

Microwaving – food is placed in a microwave oven.

Poaching – food and water are added to a pan and simmered at low heat.

Sautéing – food is prepared quickly on a high heat pan with a small amount of fat. This prevents food from sticking to the hot pan and adds flavor.

Steaming – food is placed in a bowl or steamer and cooked by steam from a small amount of water.

Stir-frying – food is prepared usually in a wok, over medium to high heat. A small amount of oil is used. The food is cut into small pieces that will cook quickly.

Task: Think about what you have eaten in the last three days. Which preparation methods did you use the most? Can you identify ways of preparing the same food in a healthier way?

———
———

———

Now we will talk about the advantages and disadvantages of these different cooking methods. Let's start with the first one.

Baking

Advantages – A wide variety of foods can be prepared and if they are prepared carefully the use of too much fat can be avoided.
Disadvantages – There is a tendency seen in some individuals to add too much fat when greasing trays and tins. This can be avoided if you use an oil spray. The timing must be right to avoid over or undercooking.

Barbecue

Advantages – This method enhances the flavor and texture of the food.
Disadvantages – Sometimes the food can be undercooked and this can lead to poor quality food or to food poisoning.

Boiling

Advantages – This method can produce stock that contains nutrients from the food that has been cooked. It can tenderize vegetables like broccoli, potato or cauliflower.
Disadvantages – Green vegetables can sometimes be overcooked when boiling is used. This can lead to them losing flavor, texture and nutrients.

Braising

Advantages – Can't tenderize cheaper, tougher cuts of meat. May improve flavor and create interesting textures.
Disadvantages – It is a slow preparation process

Casserole

Advantages – The nutrients released by the food are held in the liquid and remain available to eat. This method can tenderize cheaper cuts of meat.

Disadvantages – It is a slow preparation process that can sometimes lead to the meat being dry and overcooked.

Deep frying

Advantages – The process is quick. People often enjoy the enhanced flavors due to the cooking oils/fats.

Disadvantages – The frying process adds calories and sometimes produces cancer related chemicals. This cooking is not very healthy.

Grilling

Advantages – This method can allow fats to drain away and can seal meat and vegetables and keep in the juices. It involves less fat than the frying process.

Disadvantages – The food can be dry, or can be burned, and can release unhealthy chemicals. Grilling is not a great method to cook cheaper cuts of meat.

Microwaving

Advantages – This method is very quick. There is no need to add cooking fats and the nutrients can be kept in the food if the microwave is used with moderation.

Disadvantages – The food is often overcooked because the cooking times are so quick. It can destroy a big amount of nutrients in the food.

Poaching

Advantages – This is a good way of cooking food that would become tough if it was cooked another way. Food cooked like this is easy to digest.

Disadvantages – If the food is undercooked it is a risk of poisoning yourself.

Sautéing

Advantages – This cooking is much healthy than deep or shallow frying.

Disadvantages – Oils can burn and release bad chemicals components. It is a tendency to use too much oil/fat.

Steaming

Advantages – It is a fast method to cook fish, poultry or veg. It helps to lock in flavors and nutrients.

Disadvantages – The food can be overcooked. Red meat is unsuitable to be steamed.

Stir-frying

Advantages – This is a fast cooking method that allows the frying of food while retaining all the nutrients and is limiting the problems associated with conventional or deep frying.

Disadvantages – Food and oils can burn fast if the heat is too high.

Most of the people need to use a bigger range of cooking methods when preparing meals. This will promote variation in their diet and it will make them to experiment with different cooking styles for any different type of meals.

***

What happen if we need to prepare food? Especially if we need to prepare meals for others? If we serve food that someone does not usually include in their diet, this can potentially create health problems or we can be disrespectful of religion, beliefs and values. The questions we need to ask are:

Do you need the food to be prepared in a certain way?

Are there any food you do not like or you do not eat?

Are there any other considerations I need to know before I start cooking?

These questions can help you to find if the person has any dietary requirement due to their personal beliefs, religion or health. We also need to avoid cross contamination when we are preparing food, either by your hands or the tools you are using it.

Case study – the importance of considering other people needs when we are preparing food.

Natasha was cooking chips for herself, a vegetarian friend and a Jewish friend. Normally, Natasha would use lard (pork fat) for her chips. But her normal cooking habits would not be tolerated on this occasion. In order to make her meal suitable for a vegetarian and a Jew, she would use olive oil instead.

A diet that it is unhealthy can make people have a poorer quality of life and can develop health problems, costing them a lot of money. Despite this, many of us will continue to eat unhealthily. What are the main reasons? The conflicting information about healthy eating and diets can cause confusion and people can be not informed enough. Some people consider that healthy food is too expensive or they are leaving fresh products to go to waste. However, a research done over many decades shows that overall the cost of eating unhealthy food and the health costs related are much bigger than the cost of eating healthy meals and health costs related. Long term is better for everyone to eat healthy, economically speaking. It can be hard for some to go the large supermarkets which have a greater selection of meals, because they are sometimes outside town. Fat food and ready meals are a quicker and more convenient option, as they require less preparation. Longer working hours and busy social live can make it difficult for us to plan and prepare healthy meals.

Now let's discuss about every reason in particular.

Confusion – many people are confused or ill-informed about what healthy eating is. The media is packed with ideas about the role-models and the desire to eat healthy, but the information is often conflicting. There is always a new product claiming to change your life and a new diet which promise you amazing results fast. There is so much information that you can be overloaded by the sheer volume and the contradictory nature of what you read or hear. When faced with confused or mixed messages, it is difficult for us to make informed decisions about what we should eat. Just to give an example, a product labeled reduced fat isn't necessarily low in fat. Also, as children, we learn about diet from the adults around us, if they are ill informed, the habits we develop could be unhelpful too. If someone is ill informed, it is more likely to make poor nutritional choices.

Case study

Andrew just started work in another town and it is his first time he has lived away from home. He lives in a shared house with other colleagues and has to cook for himself. He rarely saw his parents cook for him, as they both worked full time and often ate separately. As a result, Andrew has almost no cooking skills and he doesn't like vegetables. His diet will be high in protein, fats and carbs (including ready meals, takeaways and pizza), he also has a high alcohol intake. After few months, he noticed that he is putting on some weight, but he didn't know what to do, as he never learnt what a balanced diet looked like.

What he should do?

First of all, he need to get reliable nutritional information, because familiarizing you with up to date nutritional advice is the first step towards a healthy diet. If you educate yourself about nutrition and healthy eating, those in your care are also eating healthier and you encourage a lifetime of healthy eating habits. As science advance, the nutritional advice sometimes change, so it is important to make sure that what you know is current and relevant to your circumstances. Always keep in mind from where the information is coming from. Reliable, impartial sources, as NHS website for example, are going to be more trustworthy than suggestions made in magazines or online. Products that make health claims are doing so to sell, so always check the label.

Now, Andrew used the NHS website to calculate his BMI online, and found his daily energy requirements. He also went to his local health center, where British Nutrition Foundation helps you to find what you need to eat for a balanced and healthy diet. He started to check the nutritional content of the food he was buying and to avoid the ones with high fat and sugar content. He purchased a student cook book, in order to use easy to prepare, nutritional meals.

B) Costs as a reason to not eat healthy – it is one of the most common reasons people use when we talk about healthy eating. There are always way to alleviate this, like using promotions and discounts (but the ones who live alone and are on low incomes may not use this, as the extra food can go to waste). You may think that buying organic fruit and veg is more expensive, and that frozen, ready to microwave meals are cheaper than buying the ingredients and cooking from scratch, but if you are looking at it long term, the cost of all these salty, sugary and fatty foods is very high. Being overweight, having poor skin, low energy and being prone to suffer of many illnesses as a result of having an unhealthy diet is too much to pay as you get older.

Case study

Ruby is a busy mom living on a low income. She has a 2 years old girl and twins, who are 4 years old. Ruby needs to budget everything carefully, allocating money for mortgage, bills, transport, children and food every month. She has a very strict budget for her weekly shopping, and she would like to cook more from scratch, but it is hard to find the time to do this, and she thinks that can be expensive to buy all the ingredients needed.

Facts check

Fresh ingredients are not always more expensive, especially when you need more food and buy in bulk to feed a large family. Ruby can research some meals that are quick and easy to prepare, she can look out for multi-buy offers on the ingredients that are usually used, and she can also cook in large quantities, so that she can freeze few portions for the other day. She can buy fruit and veg that are in the season, and the price for them is cheaper.

Here is a mini-strategy on how to spend less on yours 5-a-day.

-buying loose fruit and veg can be cheaper.
-buy them if they are in season for the same reason.
-eat a fruit as a snack instead of chocolate or pack of crisps, it is healthier and cheaper.
-cook in bulk and freeze some food for later.
-do not throw away you vegetables if they are going to be out of date, use them for stew of casserole and freeze them for later.
-stock up cans of fruit and veg, the better option are the ones in water or own juice, without added sugar or salt.
- look up for supermarket deals as buy one, get one free.
- swap ready-made meals for homemade alternatives, it is usually cheaper to do them for scratch.
- look for good deals of frozen fruit and veg like peas, pulses, they are cheaper than fresh ones, but still healthier than fast food.

C) Accessibility as a reason to avoid healthy choices – not everyone can go and shop for their food in a large supermarket, as they are usually on the outskirts of towns, so this can be difficult for people with limited transport options. Public transport schedule can be a problem, or time, if you are a mother with small children. If you are old, carrying heavy shopping home can be challenging. As a child or elderly who depends of others to get their shopping or cooking the meals, can be difficult to have a healthy diet if your carers insist on buying ready meals of fast food instead of cooking from scratch. Large out of town supermarkets are cheaper and have a wider range of products, but you can also use local shops such as green grocers and neighborhood butchers. But smaller shops are not only offering a limited choice of foods, they are also a bit more expensive.

CHAPTER 2
THE INDIVIDUAL NUTRITIONAL NEEDS

Nutritional needs and dietary requirements are different while we are ageing. There are three main groups of people about whom you will learn about in this chapter.

A. Young children in the age category from 1 to 4 years old, with an energy requirement of 920-1300 kcal.

Diet example:

Carbohydrates – 3 servings

1-2 slices of bread (20-80 g depending on age)
1-3 tablespoons of cornflakes (15-30 g of cereal depending on age)
1-3 tablespoon of mashed potato (30-80 g depending on age)

Protein – 2 servings

1-3 tablespoons of chopped meat or fish or tofu (20-60 g depending on age)
1-2 fish fingers/Quorn sausage

Dairy – 3 servings

1 pot of yogurt or fromage fraiche
2 cups/beakers of 120 ml milk

Fruit – 3 servings

7 strawberries or 2 plums
1 medium banana
1 large pineapple slice

Vegetables – 2 servings

1-3 heaped tablespoons of cooked veg (carrots, peas, sweet corn)
3 sticks of celery

B. Children in the age category from 5 to 12 years old, with an energy requirement of 1300-1800 kcal.

Diet example:

Carbohydrates – 4 servings

100 g of boiled potatoes is one serving

Protein – 3 servings

3-5 tablespoons of mince or finely chopped meat
2-4 fish fingers
1-2 eggs (poached or scrambled)

Dairy – 3 servings

1 cup of 120 ml milk
1 pot of yogurt
1 cheese in sandwich (40-60 g) or milk based pudding

Fruit – 2 servings

7 strawberries or 2 plums
1 banana or 1 large pineapple slice

Vegetables - 3 servings

4 heaped tablespoons of green vegetables is one serving

C. Teenagers in the age group from 13 to 18 years old, with an energy requirement of 1800-2700 kcal.

Diet example:

Carbohydrates – 5-10 servings (depending on age, gender and activity levels)

Two small boiled potatoes is one serving
3 tablespoons of breakfast cereal or boiled pasta is one serving
115 g of cooked noodles is one serving

Protein – 3 servings

75 g of cooked meat is one serving
150 g of white fish is one serving
Two medium sized eggs is one serving

Dairy – 3 servings

1 cup of 150-250 ml milk
1 pot of 150 ml yogurt
1 milk based pudding

Fruit – 3 servings

7 strawberries of 2 plums
1-2 handfuls of berries or grapes
1 banana

Vegetables – 3 servings

3 tablespoons of peas, beans or pulses
7 cherry tomatoes
8 cauliflower florets

A serving is different than a portion. Servings are recommended amounts of food, portions are defined by our choice regarding the amount of food we want to eat. Portion sizes are completely in your control, you can choose a bigger or smaller portion than the recommended serving. For example, the label of a pizza box may advise that the pizza serves 4 people, but your portion can be more or less than the recommended serving. It is very easy for children and young people to lose track or forget about the caloric and nutritional content of the food, as they may not find calorie counting very interesting. Planning the meals and the snacks in advance is the best way to help a child or a teenager to get all the nutrients needed in their diet.

Here is one example of planning. We did this for Dennis, age 6.

Breakfast
200 ml low fat milk (Dairy serving 1)
1 large slice of toast (Carbohydrates serving 1)

Snacks
200 ml low fat milk (Dairy serving 2)
1 medium banana (Fruit serving 1)

Lunch
2-4 tablespoons of mashed potatoes – 80 g, 80 g of chicken breast
(Carbohydrates serving 2, Protein serving 1)
4 tablespoons of green beans (Veg serving 1)

Snacks
100 ml of yogurt (Dairy serving 3)
1 orange (Fruit serving 2)

Dinner
Spaghetti Bolognese made with lean mince (Protein servings 2 and 3)
Sauce with grated carrot and peppers (Veg servings 2 and 3)
25 g of boiled pasta (Carbohydrates serving 3)

Why we need to do this? Children and young adults require different amounts of nutrient and calories depending of their age. If we know exactly whom your meal plan is for will make it easy for us to find their energy and nutritional requirements. Before we start a meal plan we need to know what is needed for a healthy balanced diet and work out which food and drink we will choose to provide these nutrients. Meal plans are very useful for the parents of young children to make it sure that they receive all the nutrients needed. Meal plans are also needed in schools, if children will attend a breakfast of afterschool club, because the school has a duty to provide balanced, healthy meals.

Energy requirements and how they change with age is an important subject for any parent. The amount of calories a person need in their childhood years increases continuously before reaching a plateau by the time of them being 18 years old.

For a child of 3 to 12 months old, the energy requirements increase continuously as the baby grows. While their daily amount of calories may not seem like a lot, in proportion with their body, they need to consume a bigger amount of food than other age groups.

For a child of 1 to 6 years old, the energy requirements increase steadily for both girls and boys, due to their rate of growth.

For a child of 6 to 14 years old, the required energy sees an increase, but at a slightly slower rate as the growth tails off. It is usually at this age that girls begin to require a lot less energy than boys.

For a child of 14 to 18 years old, you can see another spike in energy requirements due to growth spurts and changes in the body during puberty for both girls and boys. This is usually the point where the energy requirements hit their highest point in every person's lifespan.

For an adult of 18 years old or more, the energy requirement gradually decrease as the body stop growing and the adult become less physically active.

***

The nutritional profiles of young children

Planning a balanced diet is not just about giving to a child all the required energy. Meal plans must also ensure that the child is getting all the needed nutrients. Anyway, just like the energy requirements, the nutritional plan also changes very fast during the childhood. Children will need fewer calories than adults because they are not so big, but they are constantly growing and are very active, so the daily amount of calories is steadily increasing. Despite this, the children should have smaller portions than adults. Salt should be avoided and never be added to very young children's food, as their kidneys cannot cope with higher levels of salt. In order to avoid this, do not add gravy to a child meal, do not use stock cubes when you prepare soup or casserole for them. Fruits will have all the natural sugar a child will need in the daily diet, so sweets and sugary, fizzy drinks should be kept to a minimum. If you add processed sugar to a baby's food too early, you can build a habit of preference for sweet foods, resulting in potential health problems as the child gets older. Children under 12 months should not consume bee honey due to the risk of botulism, an illness that is potentially dangerous at this age. Milk is vital for growth and developing strong bones and teeth. Baby milk is the only food in the first 6 months, and should be given at least 600 ml daily until they are at least 12 months old. After that they can drink cow's milk, but this need to be full fat because they need the calories and the fats from it. Solid food is difficult to eat and digest and can contain extra salt. Starting to eat solid food to early will cause allergies, illness, stomach cramps and other long term damage. From 6-9 months old, they can eat mashed and finger foods like potatoes, vegetables, fruits, pieces of cheese, yogurts and strips of toast. After 9 months they can start to eat chopped meat, beans and other kind of food. A lack of vitamin D and calcium can cause rickets (a bone disease), and a lack of iron can cause anemia. If they eat too much fibre, this can cause bloating and prevent them from eating enough food. The children under age of 5 only have access to the foods they parents prepare or buy for them. Their food should be fresh, including plenty of fruit and vegetables, starchy food as potato or pasta, protein from pulses, fish or meat and wholegrain cereals. A balanced diet will not only ensure that the child is getting all the required nutrients, but will also build good eating habits that carry on into adulthood.

Let's see which foods are good sources of key ingredients. Calcium is found is milk, cheese and dairy products. Calcium rich foods list will include plain yogurt, whole grain bread, and cheese as ricotta or cheddar.

Iron can be found in beans, leafy green vegetables and red meat such as beef, pork and lamb. You can add to you diet sources of iron like broccoli, fortified cereals or lean meat.

Good sources of vitamin A include cheese, eggs, carrots, yogurt and low fat spreads.

Fruit and vegetables are rich in vitamin C, you need to include in your diet peppers, oranges, blackcurrants, strawberries, potatoes and broccoli.

Vitamin D is coming mainly from sunlight, but can be also found in oily fish, eggs and fortified cereals.

Good sources of protein for children are: peanut butter, milk, and cheese and turkey breast.

Carbohydrates need to be 50-60% of a child daily nutritional intake. Good sources of carbs are: brown rice, wholegrain cereals and breads, fresh fruit and veg.
Fats found in junk and fast food are unhealthy and should be avoided, however there are good sources of fat as trout, salmon, peanut butter, nuts and milk that can be used.

***

Now we will find out what are the most common nutrient deficiencies and why. Iron deficiency is one of the most common in England. The National Diet and Nutrition Survey of 2009 found that 27% of teenage girls and 13% of teenage boys have low iron levels. Active lifestyle, combined with poor diet and rapid growth, will have iron deficiency anemia as a result. Vitamin D is essential for growth, strong bones and good health. A lack of vitamin D will cause rickets in children and osteomalacia in adults. Calcium intake bellow the recommended level was found in 25% of teens, during a recent research. This can have serious implications for their future bone health. As for older people, low calcium intake can cause brittle and weak bones, a significant root of many of their health problems.

Let's explore this questions a bit more. We consider an imaginary situation off a small nursery starting in August, with accommodation provided for seven girls. They are all 2-3 years old. After her inquest, the nursery manager found that four of them have moderate activity levels and they will need 1220 calories per day. The other three girls are more active and they will need 1450 calories per day. They asked a nutritionist to advise them on the servings of the food needed by the children and for some sample menus to help them to learn what to prepare. The nutritionist gave them the following advice for each group of children, related to what they should eat, depending on their energy requirements.

For the 1200 calories/day group
Carbohydrates 4 servings/115 g
Protein 3 servings/85 g
Milk 2 servings/2 cups
Fruit 2 servings
Vegetables 3 servings

For the 1400 calories/day group
Carbohydrates 5 servings/140 g
Protein 4 servings/115 g
Milk 2 servings/2 cups
Fruit 3 servings
Vegetables 3 servings

Now, three of the girls who need 1200 calories/day are vegetarian. Everybody else will eat meat and fish. The nursery will probably need to provide meals for the children.

Menu sample – 1200 kcal/day, non-vegetarian

Breakfast
Slice of toast with boiled egg

Snack
Small carrot sticks or grated

Lunch
Turkey breast sandwich (45 g) with 2 thin slices of wholemeal bread and lettuce
2 spears of broccoli, small, chopped
120 ml of semi-skimmed milk

Snack
1 little pot of fromage fraiche
1 normal sized apple, diced

Dinner
Jacket potato with 25 g grated cheese, sweet corn and tuna
100 ml of natural fresh juice

Menu sample – 1200 kcal/day, vegetarian

Breakfast
Blueberry pancake (25-35 g)
100 ml of semi-skimmed milk

Snack
Two small Satsuma

Lunch
Veggie burger with one large wholemeal bun
100 ml of semi-skimmed milk

Snack
1 pot of fromage fraiche

Dinner
Vegetable and butter bean risotto
Mixed salad

2.1 Nutritional requirements of a child

Everyone who reaches their teens will usually have a growth spurt, this is the age when the children gain 50% of their adult weight and 20% of their adult height. Because the change and growth is increasing dramatically, the needs for all nutrients also increase. Calcium and iron intake is very important at this age. The emphasis should be on creating and maintaining good eating habits, to avoid skipping meals or eating too much junk food (high in saturated fats and sugar). Due to all the activity and growth, teenagers need 2500-3000 calories per day if they are boys, 2200-2500 per day as girls. It is best to have a diet with lean protein, low fat dairy, whole grains, fruits and vegetables. Iron helps to carry oxygen around the body, and a deficiency of it can lead to anemia, weakness and fatigue. Boys need approx. 8-11 mg/day, girls need 15 mg, due to menstruation. You can provide enough iron if you eat eggs, wholegrain foods, green vegetables, fish and meat. Hydration is very important for active young people and they should drink plenty of fluids, such as milk, fruit juice or water. Alcoholic drinks, fizzy and sugary drinks and coffee will dehydrate rather than hydrate the human body.

Salt is an nutritional factor that we need to monitor closely. Starting from th age of 11 years onwards, the maximum recommended daily intake is 6 grams per day. The teenagers need 45-55 g or protein/day, in order to grow and maintain muscle. You can easily get this eating dairy, fish and meat, if you are vegetarian you need to have your daily protein intake from sources like soy products, nuts, pulses and beans. If you do not get enough calcium as a teen, you may have weak bones and osteoporosis later in life. The recommended intake for teenagers is 800-1000 mg. As an adult you will need only 700 mg, most of it coming from cereals and dairy.

Case study

Paul

Paul is a 16 years old and has found lately that he needs to eat more in order to feel full. Because he is struggling to adapt to this increase in his energy requirements, he is often snacking of unhealthy sweets and energy bars and find hard to resist fast food when he is going out.

Nuts and seeds – Yes
Paul can snack on nuts and seeds instead of chocolate bars.

Bread and pasta – Not really
Bread and pasta are filling, but wholegrain will be a better choice. Bread can be also providing extra salt.

Water – Yes
Paul can just confuse his thirst for hunger. He needs to be properly hydrated.

Cereals – Maybe
Breakfast cereals are good, but some of them are high in sugar, so he cannot eat too much.

Paul's meal plan
Luckily for Paul his brother is a dietician, so he asks him to put together a meal plan for him. This is the result.

Breakfast
Fresh fruit smoothie with milk (Dairy serving no. 1, fruit serving no. 1)
Scrambled eggs with wholegrain toast (Carbs servings 1-2, Protein serving 1)

Snack
Cucumber and carrot sticks (Veg serving 1)

Lunch
Rice and bean enchiladas with spring onions, salad, salsa, yogurt and cheese (Carbs serving 3, protein serving 2, veg serving 2, dairy serving 2)

Snack
Natural yogurt and 6 sliced strawberries (Dairy serving 3, fruit serving 2)

Dinner
Chicken breast – 115 g – two boiled potatoes, asparagus and green beans (Protein serving 3, carbs servings 4-5, veg servings 3-4)

Remember that every one of us has an eating pattern, what we eat, when we eat and where we eat. Some are very strict with 3 meals per day and no snacks, others may snack when is needed and never plan their meals. Young children are usually very active with lots of energy to burn off. Their high activity demands a higher level of calories despite their small bodies. Children are influenced by their parents and the other adults around them. Adults decide where and when family eat, at the table or in the front of TV.

Children can make food choices, but the people cooking for them are the ones who decide what they eat. The working pattern of their parents will influence when the children eat, who they eat with and whether it is the same every day. The children may eat home cooked healthy meals every day or be exposed early to processed food, depending on their parent's food preference. They need some essential nutrients in their diet regularly, the list of them being: calcium, iron, protein, carbs and fats, vitamin A, C and D. They need all those nutrients in order to grow and give to their bodies what is needed. But we need not to forget that everyone has different eating habits and there are different factors which may affect someone's eating pattern.

Case study

Andrea and Violet

Andrea, age 4, lives with her mom, 2 brothers and a sister. She is in the same class with Violet and they are best friends. When she comes home from the school, Andrea plays in the garden with her siblings, or inside the house, creating fun games, if it is raining.

Violet, age 4, lives with her parents who have a shift based work. The often have alternate working patterns, with one working on night shifts and the other working days. Violet is in her second year of pre-school and has also started gymnastics classes. She eats her breakfast of organic cereals and a glass of milk every day, with her brother Aidan.

Andrea's mum is an acclaimed writer who works from home. She earns a lot of money which influences the range and types of food she buys for her children. She enjoys cooking and is often experimenting varied meals. As a family, they always eat in front of their favorite TV show, and Andrea likes to have a glass of milk before going to bed.

Violet eats her dinner at 5 pm, or later is she has a gymnastics class. One of her parents will cook the meal, though neither of them thinks at this as an enjoyable experience. As they don't have much time for food shopping or is they just come of work, they might go out for dinner or order a takeaway.

Think about 10 ways to improve Andrea and Violet diets. What is the reasoning behind your choices?

2.2 Nutritional needs of a teenager

They are growing fast, so they will get hungry often and need extra calories. A teenager needs to adapt his diet to their lifestyle. One who is exercising regularly will have a different diet than another teenager who does little to none physical activity. At this age you have far more independence over what and when you eat, because of a busy schedule and having your own money. It was determined that as they get older, the teenagers are more likely to skip breakfast and choose a lie-in instead. To plan a better eating pattern you need to ask if they are eating with family or alone, how healthy is theirs food, if they like to snack and what they eat at that time, if they stay up and eat late or if they drink alcohol and how much.

What about planning meals for older people? What are the nutritional needs when you are doing this, even if you can apply the same basic principles, variety and balance? Well, the emphasis should be of good eating habits. But there are some minor differences. When you are old, you may not drink enough fluids to satisfy your body need for hydration. It is needed to drink at least 8 glasses of fluid daily, more if you are doing any kind of exercise. Vitamins B (B6, B12 and folic acid) are very important for their health and wellbeing. Sources of folic acid are fruits and vegetables, B12 can be found on fortified cereals and meat, B6 can be found in cereals, beans fish and some fruits and veg. As you get older, you start to lose bone mass, so calcium rich foods are very important. As you are more prone to osteoporosis ((losing bone mass, by losing an excessive amount of protein, mineral content and calcium), you need to start to eat more milk, yogurt, cheese, tuna and salmon, to manage it, often without any need for medication. Salt intake for older people should be lesser than 6 g per day. As you start to have a reduced sense of taste, you may try to compensate for this by adding salt. Calories decline as you get older. At age of 59, you may need 2250 calories as a male and 1950 as e female. At 64, you may need only 2375 calories as a male and 1900 as a woman. At 75 or older, males will need less than 2100, and females less than 1800. As people get old, their physical power diminish, heart become slower, arteries stiffen, bones shrink in size and density, muscles lose strength and flexibility, coordination diminishes and eyesight may worsen. They will have lower levels of activity and lower energy requirements as a result if ageing. As opposes to the time when they are employed, when their daily work routine will involve some physical activity, as people retire, their activity levels will fall significantly, and so will their energy requirements. Despite the general expectation that older people become less active as they retire (reflected by the compulsory retirement age imposed by law or the stereotype of elderly walking with sticks of using a wheelchair), we are slowly changing, and now older people are encouraged to increase their physical activity when it is possible. But generally, as a result of retirement, they will eat fewer calories than a healthy adult. They need to try to keep active and to understand that eating less does not necessarily lead to loss of the essential nutrients. They can have fewer calories, but they will still need to sustain a healthy, varied and balanced diet. People over 65 need less energy than teenagers and adults, but more than the children.

If their diet will be poor, they can suffer from malnutrition. Let's talk about some of the potential causes of this risk. If someone prepares meals for an elderly, they might not understand their nutritional needs. They might not know how to cook the meals that the other person enjoys or they can prepare it in a way the older person does not like it. If you are old, you may eat most of all of your meals alone. When people eat in social groups, they may eat more and take care to choose wholesome, healthy meals. Conditions such as dementia can make an elderly to forget what or if they have eaten. Physical infirmity can prevent shopping, food preparation or even make it difficult to feed themselves. If they suffer from depression, they may not feel like preparing or eating at all. Some medication can also suppress the appetite. Some people who live alone may have limited understanding of shopping, balanced food preparation and cooking, especially if they lived with others who took responsibility for shopping and cooking. The person who went through separation may have little knowledge of nutrition or cooking. If they have lower incomes, they may find convenient to buy cheaper ready meals with limited nutritional value and prepare less food from scratch. Some older people can find difficult to get access to shops that offer a bigger range of nutritious foods, in order to have a balanced diet. With so many factors potentially leading to malnutrition and impacting diet, it is necessary that the eating habits of an older people.

Case study

Suggested meal plan for Brian, age 66

Early morning

Tea of coffee with semi-skimmed milk
(Dairy serving 1)

Breakfast

Toast, butter and jam
(Carbs serving 2)

Snack
Medium sized banana
(Fruit serving 1)

Lunch

Poached salmon with sweet potatoes, green beans and asparagus
Yogurt with strawberries
(Protein serving 1, carbs servings 2&3, veg servings 1&2, dairy serving 2,
fruit serving 2)

Snack

Rice pudding
(Carbs serving 4)

Evening meal

Jacket potatoes with tuna salad
(Veg serving 3, carbs serving 5, protein serving 2)

Snack

Hot drink – Tea, milk, Ovaltine, hot chocolate
With biscuits
(Dairy serving 3)

Their daily intake should generally follow this rule:
Fruit and veg – 5 servings
Carbs – 5 servings
Dairy – 3 servings
Protein – 2 servings

Fatty and sugary foods – not too much.

Most common problems for elderly people are constipation and digestive problems (a fibre rich diet can help to prevent this), osteoporosis (especially for women, leading to fractures, eating enough calcium and vitamin D can help, however having too much vitamin A can worsen things), less energy (caused by an iron deficiency).

***

When we talk about nutritional requirements, we need also to talk about special dietary needs. There are a number of factors affecting a person, who might have special dietary requirements: related to health are allergies, intolerances and health conditions, related to religious reasons are ethnic groups and religious beliefs, personal reasons as lifestyle and moral values. Allergies will make someone body immune system particularly sensitive to some foods, that can cause an allergic reaction. They need to avoid this kind of food. If you are allergic to a food the reaction could be minimal such as mouth irritation, but in some cases can lead to anaphylactic shock, life threatening if it is not dealt quickly. Common allergies include nuts, wheat, fish and shellfish. Some people carry an EpiPen in case they come in contact with the food they are allergic at it. Young children are also often allergic to egg and soy. Intolerance is the phenomenon that causes the body to be unable to properly digest certain foods. It is longer before a reaction occurs than for an allergy, but the symptoms may last longer too. Enzymes are needed to digest food. If some of the enzymes are missing, the body may not be able to properly digest certain foods. Common intolerance includes lactose (dairy and milk), beans, cabbage and citrus fruit. They need to avoid this food. Coeliac disease and diabetes are conditions which demand specific diets. Coeliacs are unable to eat gluten products. Those suffering from diabetes will have to limit their sugar intake. Certain ethnic groups and religions have strict beliefs about what cannot be eaten. People belonging to these groups will have diets that follow these rules. Some people will choose a specific diet for moral or personal reasons. Like someone who choose to not eat meat because they believe that killing animals for food is wrong. Coeliac disease is commonly referred as gluten intolerance, but it is not intolerance, nor an allergy. The body immune system mistakes gluten for something threatening and attacks it, damaging the surface of the small intestine and affecting the ability to absorb nutrients. People with coeliac disease need to avoid gluten food at all cost (such as bread, cake, biscuits, pizza, pasta, cereal, sauces or ready meals, beer, lager and ale). Diabetes occurs when glucose is not transformed in energy, because we do not have enough insulin or it doesn't work properly (sugar level in the body is controlled by insulin hormone, which removes glucose from the blood and take it into cells where is transformed in energy). There are two types of them, diabetes type 1, where our immune system attacks the cells that produce insulin, so we will not have enough insulin to convert glucose into energy, and diabetes type 2, where our body does not react to insulin or does not produce enough insulin. Type one will be controlled with insulin injections, type 2 will be controlled with a limited carbohydrates diet and medication. Talking about religious groups, if a person belongs to one, this can have a significant influence of their alimentary preferences. Let's see! For Jews, pork and shellfish products are forbidden and any other meat must be killed in a specific way (Kosher). They do not eat milk and meat together and utensils must be kept separate, they also fast at certain times during the year, most important being Yom Kippur. They can drink alcohol, as long as it is made with kosher ingredients. Sikh do not drink alcohol and eat beef, some of them are vegetarian or avoid meat killed in a kosher or halal way. They may fast during full moon or on certain dates. Hindus are not usually eating meat, fish, poultry or eggs. When they eat meat, they will avoid beef or any leftover food. Muslim are avoiding pork, carrion and blood, any other meat must be killed in a specific way (called Halal). They are forbidden to eat any product containing pork fat or non-halal meat or animal fat. Gelatin also needs to be Halal. They do not drink alcohol and fast during the month of Ramadan. Buddhists have no food restrictions, but many may choose to be vegetarian. Some Buddhists are vegetarian, some vegan, some will avoid garlic, onion, leek, mushrooms, alcohol and caffeine. Christian eats any kind of food, and fast at certain times. In many religions they pray or thank God for the food. Fasting it is also important , Buddhists fast completely on certain days, Christians have many fasting days during the year, Lent being important, Hindus got 18 major holidays that may include feasting or fasting, some Hindu will also fast on the anniversaries of the death of their parents, during the Ramadan, Muslims are not allowed to eat between sunrise and sunset. Jews fast in a number of days, most common being called Passover. Belonging to an ethnic group will also influence what a person does and doesn't eat. The food is mostly affected by the climate and soils from a specific region, so isolate communities will eat the fruits, vegetables and meat that are growing local, with little or no exposure to other new foods. If you are familiar with specific foods, you may want to eat according to your ethnic or cultural background, but now we are exposed to a wide range of cultures, offering a wider range of different foods. Now, that we are able to transport food and ingredients quickly and easily, we can have access to food originated from all over the world.

Vegetarians choose to not eat meat because of their values and beliefs. There are many kinds of vegetarian diet. Vegetarian in the accepted way, will avoid meat, fish, shellfish and animal products, main motivation being the ethical concern about harming the animals. Demi-vegetarians will eat meat occasionally, but their primary food is vegetarian. Pescetarians will have a vegetarian diet, but they will add fish for its Omega 3 content and essential fatty oils. Lacto-ovo-vegetarians are most common in the Western world, they will add dairy and eggs. Lactovegetarians will eat dairy products, but not eggs (very popular in the East – Hindu, Sikh and Buddhists). Ovo-vegetarians will not eat milk, but they will use free range eggs from non-caged hens. Fruitarians will eat only foods that are harvested without killing the host plant (fruits falling from the tree). Vegans will avoid all animal related products, not only foods. Raw vegans will have the same diet like vegans, but only uncooked. People become vegetarians for various reasons, health problems, they do not like meat or believe that it is healthier to eat like this or they believe that killing animals in order to eat them is wrong. Vegetarians and vegans need to be careful with their diet, in order to provide all the essential nutrients.

Case study

Ms. Smith son, John, has become a raw vegan while at university. Before the summer holiday, Ms. Smith made a list of foods that John would no longer eat. Then she did a research to find out how they could be replaced.

She collected the following information:

No milk, cheese and yogurt (Missing nutrient: Calcium – strong bones and teeth)
Alternative sources: dried fruit, pulses, sesame seeds.

Missing nutrient: Vitamin D (helps Calcium absorption)
Alternative sources: sunshine, fortified cereals and fat spreads.

No red meat (Missing nutrient: Iron – essential for the production of red cells)
Alternative sources: dark green veg, nuts, wholemeal bread.

Missing nutrient: Vitamin B 12 (healthy blood and nervous system)
Alternative sources: fortified cereals, fortified soy milk, yeast extract spreads.

Oily fish (Missing nutrient: Omega 3 fatty acids – healthy heart and reducing the risk of health disease)
Alternative sources: walnuts, linseed or flaxseed oil, tofu.

***

Let's speak a bit about preparing food for others. There are many factors that can determine what a person does and doesn't eat. If one is served a meal that it is not usually in his diet, this can potentially have serious consequences such as being disrespectful or beliefs, values or religion and health problems like allergies. If you are preparing food for another person, these are the questions you need to be asking about their diet:

Is there any consideration that I need to take into account?
Are there any foods you do not like or you do not eat?
Do you need your food to be prepared in a certain way?

With these questions you can determine if the person has any dietary requirements due to their religion, personal beliefs or health. When you prepare food for more than one person, you need to be careful with your hands and your utensils, to avoid cross contamination. Now let's have one example why it is important to keep other's needs in mind at all times while preparing food.

Case study

Hannah is cooking chips for herself, a vegetarian and a Jewish friend. Normally, she will fry her chips in lard (pork fat). She realizes that her normal cooking habits are not acceptable on this occasion, so Hannah decides to use rapeseed oil instead.

***

There are barriers to healthy eating that prevent people to have a balanced diet. Information overload and contradictory and confusing advices, costs or accessibility, pre-prepared and fast food are just a few of the reasons of an unhealthy diet, leading to a poorer quality of life and health problems as you get older. Now we will talk about each of them in particular, to see how we can avoid making these mistakes.

A) Confusion – the amount of conflicting information about how to eat healthy and have a balanced diet can result in people being ill-informed. This can be a result of the advertising and product information that we see around us. Media is packed with ideas about how we need to look and how to eat healthy, but the information is often conflicting and confusing, often without properly explaining why something is good for you. Some diets recommend eating less carbs, others recommend eating only carbs, and so on. There is always some new extra-healthy product or some new diet or weight loss regimen promising fast and excellent results. This could also lead to information overload, due to the sheer volume of the information and its contradictory nature. If you are faced with mixed or confusing messages, can be difficult for you to make an informed choice about your diet. For example, just because a product is labeled reduced fat, this doesn't mean that the product is low in fat. We learn from the people around us too, so young people can often pick unhealthy eating habits from their parents (if you believe that a bag of crisps and a fizzy drink is a normal breakfast, you will do that choice as an adult too.

Case study

Solomon is starting a job in London and it is the first time he has lived away from his home. He lives in a shared accommodation with other colleagues and has to cook for himself. Solomon rarely saw his parents cooking for him, as they were working full time in shifts and most of the time they ate separately. He got almost no cooking skills and he does not like vegetables. His diet is high in protein, fats and carbs, including lots of fast food, pizza and takeaways and he also has a high alcohol intake. Few months later, Solomon was putting on some extra weight, but he did not know what to change, since he never learnt what a healthy and balanced diet looked like.

Task: Do you think Solomon's diet is unhealthy? How can he improve it?

____

____

____

Sometimes you need to learn about up-to-date nutritional advice, especially if you are a parent or carer for the old and infirm. Educating yourself about nutrition and healthy eating means that those in your care will also benefit from it. If you have children, you will encourage them to create and maintain healthy eating habits. With all this ongoing research and scientific advances, the nutritional advice can sometimes change, so it is important to make sure that the information that you use is current and relevant to you and your circumstances. Yu need to check from where the information is coming from. Impartial sources such as the NHS website or British Nutrition Foundation are more reliable that articles in magazines or online media, just to give an example.

Back to Solomon, let's see how he overcame his confusion about his diet and his nutritional requirements. He used the NHS website BMI calculator to check his energy requirements. He went to his local health center and asked for guidance, trying to find out what food he need to eat for a healthy, balanced diet. When he was out shopping, he started to check the label and remained suspicious of products that made claims about reduced sugar of fat contents too. He even purchased a student cook book, full of easy to prepare healthy meals.

B) Costs – some consider healthy, organic foods to be too expensive or buy too much fresh products that often go to waste. But this is not always true. You can use promotions and discounts, but they are not very beneficial if you live alone or you are on low income, because multibuy and buy 1-get 1 free promotions will lead to extra food going to waste. It is a common belief that healthy eating is expensive and fast food is cheap. Yes, it is true that organic fruits and vegetables are more expensive, and takeaways and frozen meals are cheaper than buying all the ingredients required making a meal, but if you are thinking on long term, the added cost for your health is very high. Becoming overweight, having poor skin, low energy and being prone to suffer from different illnesses it is very often too much to pay for the commodity of eating cheaper convenience meals and fast food.

John is a busy single father on low income. He has a 2-year old child and twins who are 4-years old. He carefully budgets everything working out how much he need to pay for mortgage, bills, transport, children and food every month. He has a very strict budget to spend on his weekly shop. He would love to cook more from scratch, but because of the small children, he find it difficult to have enough time to do it and he thinks that buying all the ingredients that he would need can be expensive.

Fact check – When you are cooking for a large family, fresh, organic and healthy ingredients are not necessarily more expensive, especially when you are buying in bulk.

Fact check
John can research for meals that are quick and easy to prepare. Look out for offers to stock up on ingredients that he can use often, and buy them when they are cheaper. Make up large quantities so he can freeze few portions to avoid cooking every day. Purchase vegetables and fruit that are in season.

Following this line of reasoning, here are few tips to have your 5 a day cheaper:
- buy fruit and veg loose, not pre-packed, as they are less expensive
- cook more and freeze few portions for later
- fruit and veg are cheaper if they are in season
- stock up canned fruit and veg, in water or own juice, without added salt or sugar (you can buy them when they are on offer)
- buy your fruits and vegetables from farmers market instead of supermarket
- eat homemade meals instead of ready-made alternatives. It is often cheaper to cook them for scratch in most of the cases.
- eat a fruit as snack when you feel hungry, it is healthier and cheaper than chocolate or chips.
- vegetables close to be out of date, use them for stews or casseroles and freeze them.
- buy frozen fruits and veg if you are on the budget, they are often cheaper than the fresh ones.
- watch for offers like 1+1 free or multibuy, but do not buy fresh fruit or veg for more than two days stock, you do not want them to go to waste.

C) Accessibility – it can be difficult for some categories of people to get to large supermarkets, for a greater selection of meals. Not everyone has the choice of where and when to do their shopping. Your circumstances or the place where you live are strongly affecting your ability to make healthy food choices. Most of the large supermarkets are placed now on the outskirts of towns, reducing the accessibility for a significant segment of population. These stores have a wider range of products, but it is difficult to go to shop there if you have limited transport options. Many hypermarkets do not have public transport serving them, but even if they have, can be difficult for a mother with small child or for an elderly to take the bus to go for shopping, carrying heavy bags home. It is also a problem to have access to healthy food if you are an young child or an elderly, and you depend on others to get your shopping and to cook your meals. Imagine how difficult it is for a child to eat healthy, if the parents insist on buying ready meals and fast food. Anyway, even if large out of town shops have a wider and cheaper choice of food, sometimes it is a good idea to check your local green grocers and independent butchers. If you can go only to nearby smaller convenience shops, they are not only expensive, but also offer only a limited choice of healthy options. They are usually getting time-saving options and limited range of fresh fruit and veg. You will always have the online shopping option, with a huge choice and home delivery, but if you are older, using a computer can be difficult for you.

Case study

Anita lives alone and it is in her late seventies. She is mobile, but cannot walk long distances. She cannot drive and she found it hard to use the bus when carrying stuff such as shopping bags. She prefers to use the local village shop, which is very close to her home, and if she goes there twice a week she has not too much to carry. However, she finds it expensive and she has a limited choice of healthy meals, so she needs to make a trip to the nearby town to buy in bulk from the large supermarket. She can find a lot of healthy options there, but the 40 minutes trip with the bus is very tiring for her. Anita finds difficult to navigate in the hypermarket due to its narrow aisles, high shelves and deep freezers.

Task: Identify any factors preventing Anita's access to healthy and nutritious food.

____

____

____

____

Did you mention?
- her age
- that she lives alone
-that she is frail and cannot carry lots of shopping
-that she cannot drive
-that she is restricted by the food of the local shop
- that she finds difficult to access the large supermarket in a nearby town?

Very often, a limited access to healthy and nutritious food and drinks is out of the hands of an individual. While some may be able to shop around for the food needed for a balanced diet, there are others that rely on friends and family to provide them with a healthiest range of food. The easy access to online food shopping means that you can still enjoy a wider range and selection of products while you are not living near large out of town supermarkets. Also, some shops are better for certain items than others. Spreading your shopping over a few different supermarkets, if it is possible, will gave you the choice of a wide and cheaper range of products. Some communities run initiatives as food cooperatives, where few people come together to buy in bulk from suppliers to make good quality food more affordable. Anyone can set up a food cooperative and provide a valuable service to his community, if the choice of food is limited in your area. There are also meals at home services (sometimes known as 'Meals of wheels'), where pre-prepared nutritious meals are delivered directly at home for old, housebound or people with disabilities, ensuring those at risk will get a healthy, nutritious and balanced diet. Recently we have more options that in the past, with the increased pressure on stores and restaurants to provide healthy alternatives and the internet online shopping, but there are still people with no access to these alternatives.

D) Convenience – fast food and ready meals are a quicker option and they require little preparation. The pre-packed meal industry in UK is worth 2.7 billion pounds, and these meals rise in popularity, despite the poor nutritional value. We are spending longer at work and less time shopping and cooking, and this entire subtle shift in perception will make us think that we do not have enough time. A meal that can be grabbed on the way back from work, fast cooked in the microwave and eaten out from the same container, with no washing up can make us believe that we save effort and time. We live in an era where we have more money and less time, and people earning much, but with not enough spare time, will see this option as a perfect compromise. Another reason can be that many of us do not know how to cook or don't enjoy it doing it. So, we will choose a ready-meal that look familiar, as we got a large variety available, even if they are not as healthy as the homemade ones. It is easier for a shop to provide convenience food with a longer shelf life rather than fresh perishable fruit, veg and meat. The taste of this kind of food seems better, because of the high level of sugar, salt and additives.

Case study

Roberta is a single woman who lives alone and commutes for 70 minutes to work every day. She does not have any cooking skills and she does not enjoy cooking. Roberta earns a good wage and she can afford to eat any kind of food she wants. Usually she buys her weekly meals and stores them in her modern freezer, having the choice to eat what she like and not spending too much time cooking it. She enjoys her meals and find this convenient. Roberta doesn't see anything wrong with this kind of diet.

Task: Can you think of any ways to improve Roberta's diet? Write your ideas bellow:

____

____

____

____

E) Lifestyle – working in shifts or having a busy social live can be an obstacle in planning and cooking healthy meals. There is a whole new attitude of eating on the move, especially for the ones commuting with the train, for example. You can see it often, doing emails, eating and having a drink you his/her way to work. This has resulted in a wider range of fast foods and convenience food meals that can be made quickly to maximize your spare time. People travel more nowadays, so they develop a taste for food that they have never seen cooked and appears to be much easier to buy it than to try to cook it from scratch. Sadly, the new generations of children grow up without seeing their parents cooking healthy food, and most probably they will follow them and do the same as they grow up.

Case study

Eleanor and Daniel are young professionals working in the City and living nearby. They usually buy a coffee and a croissant on the way to work, they are also eating lunch with clients very often and because they are working late, they don't have time to eat at home before their evening plans. Having a busy social life, they pick some fast food on the way to cinema or theatre. They have a decent income, but not too much time to spare. When Eleanor and Daniel are at home, they find that there is not much food in the fridge, so they treat themselves with a takeaway meal.

For most of the people, there is more than one barrier to stop you from having a healthy, balanced diet. These kind of barriers can lead to bad eating habits that are very difficult to unlearn and can influence more than one generation. If you eat pre-prepared meals and fast food, this is most of the times the result of a chosen lifestyle. In order to overcome these barriers, you need to make some changes towards a healthy diet, and you may think at this as a major challenge, but in reality it is not. A group of small changes, following each other, is an effective strategy.

Let's go back to Eleanor and Daniel. They want to eat healthier, so they set up some changes to their normal routine. Sunday, when they have a day off, they will plan the meal for the next week and the ingredients they need to buy to cook it. They will prepare some extra portions and freeze them. They will wake up a bit early than usual so they have enough time to prepare some healthy lunch packs to avoid eating on the move. They went to buy long-life foods as frozen peas, tins of fruit, cans of tuna, so they can still eat a nutritious meal if it happens to run out of fresh food.

Regardless of your chosen lifestyle, you can always benefit from decreasing the amount of convenience food from your diet, eating with your family, trying to have smaller portions and planning in advance and cooking your own meal.

CHAPTER 3
PLANNING A HEALTHY DIET

In order to achieve the previous goal, we need to understand the food labels, to learn about the daily amounts of nutrients in every adult diet, to calculate how much energy is provided by the carbohydrate, protein and fat from the food and to know how to avoid misleading food label claims and descriptions. We will also learn about food additives and E-numbers, what they do and what the lawful approach for this problem is. In the end we will see how to analyze and evaluate a diet according to a healthy eating perspective and how and why we need to keep a food diary. You are familiar that we can find labels of every product purchased from the shop. It is a legal requirement for all the food and drink to carry one of this nutritional information labels, and, if you go to a supermarket, you will see a high number of different foods, many of them processed and pre-prepared, and a wide variety of ingredients. They need to be labeled to help you make decisions about them. You need to know this in order to make sensible judgments about the nutritional value of the food, to decide if I am healthy or unhealthy. In order to do this, the food needs to be labeled properly. According to the Food Labeling Regulations from 1996, the manufactured and processed foods in UK must be labeled by law.

The front labeling must show the name of the food, the expiration date or where to find it, quantity, any warning (example: Contains traces of nuts – Not suitable for people who are allergic to nuts), a list of ingredients, the name and the address of the manufacturer, packer or seller, the batch or lot number, any special storage conditions, cooking instructions if necessary. Certain products must show the country of origin (example: Produced in Italy), for products like beef, veal, shellfish, fish, honey, olive oil, vine, fruits and veg, or poultry if it is from outside the EU. There are some exceptions to these rules. In UK, food that is sold loose does not have to comply with many labeling regulations, unless is genetically modified. Nutrition labeling is optional, but become compulsory if the product makes a nutritional claim. What means nutritional claim? This means that the product has a specific nutritional property as a result of the ingredients or additives the food does or does not contain (for example: low fat, low sugar, high fiber). If a nutritional claim is made, the manufacturer must provide relevant nutritional information. If nutritional information is needed, the label must show clearly the energy value in both kilojoules (kJ) and kilocalories (kcal), the amount of carbohydrates, protein and fat in grams, value is given per 100 g or 100 ml, per package or per portion. It also must have any additional information related to the nutritional claim being made, if it was not already covered by the previous informations. A health claim is a statement or suggestion that a link exists between food and health, and that food can improve a person's health in a specific way (example: helps reduce digestive discomfort or helps support immunity). The claims need to be truthful and honest, not to mislead the consumers, must be clear and easy to understand. The effect made I the claim must be understandable to the average consumer. When promoting a food or ingredient, not attempt should be made to question the safety of nutritional value of other foods.

Reference intakes

Reference intakes – RI , previously known as Guideline Daily Amounts – GDA, were introduced by government to provide simple reliable information of food and nutrition. They tell to the consumer how much is considered a healthy amount to eat. Most of the labels will have reference intakes for an adult person on the pack. They were made simpler than GDA, and there is an only one setoff value for an adult.

Example

Saturated fat Salt

| 2.8 g | 1.35 g | per 100 g |
| 5.1 g | 2.45 g | per pizza |

| 20 g | 6 g | RI |
| 26% | 41% | per pizza |

All the information for RI will be provided in grams or diminutives of grams, except energy, measured in kilojoules – kJ, or kilocalories – kcal. As I said before, there is only one list for the energy and selected nutrients for adults.

Energy 8400 kJ / 2000 kcal

Fat   70 g
From which saturated fat 20 g

Carbohydrates 260 g
From which sugars 90 g

Protein 50 g

Salt 6 g

The RI for an adult are based on the requirements for average female with no special dietary restrictions and assumed energy intake of 2000 kcal.

There are some types of claim that are not permitted of the food labels. These are medicinal claims about prevention, treatment or curing of a disease, nutritional claims of alcoholic beverages with more than 1.2% alcohol, claims that health could be affected by not consuming that food, references to any rate or amount of weight loss as a direct result of consuming the product, references to recommendations by individual doctors / health professionals, references that are questioning the safety or nutritional content of other foods.

Case study

In May 2014 a new diet chocolate, Thin-a-lot, was released by Europe Diet Supplements Ltd. They made various claims about how effective the chocolate is as an aid in weight loss and what are the changes induced in our metabolism. The pack and the internet website of this supplement product has a signed recommendation written by a Dr. Stephen Vincent Strange making claims that those who are not eating this particular chocolate put themselves at risk of suffering heart problems. It was also a guarantee that everyone who eats it as breakfast for a three week period will lose at least 2 stones. These claims were investigated by the Advertising Standards Agency and the product was found breaching regulations outlined in the Food Labeling Regulations 1996. By November 2014 has been removed from the shops.

Task: In how many ways do you think this supplement breached the Food Labeling Regulations?

____

____

____

____

But how will you monitor your daily intake? The most important bit when you are having a healthy diet is monitoring the daily amount of fat, sugar and salt. What you need to avoid and what to include when you are trying to eat healthy? A food is high in fat if it has more than 17 g fat / 100 g, and it is low in fat if it has less than 3 g fat /100 g. A food is high in salt if it has more than 1.5 g salt / 100 g, and it is low in salt if it has less than 0.1-0.3 g / 100 g. A food is high in sugar if it has more than 22 g / 100 g, and it is low in sugar if it has less than 5 g / 100 g. You can also calculate the amount of energy by looking at the label and check the amount of carbohydrates, protein and fat and use the energy consumption informations to make the calculations.

Case study - Marian's chocolate

Marian has a chocolate as a snack. She wants to calculate the energy of the chocolate using the informations about the amount of carbohydrates, protein and fat. The product label state that one chocolate contains:

Fat 1.0 g
Protein 12.5 g
Carbohydrates 22.25 g

We have the calories from the fat 1 x 9 = 9, from the protein 12.5 x 4 = 50, from the carbohydrates 22.25 x 4 = 89, so the total amount will be 9 + 50 + 89 = 148 calories.

Another example – half a can of pasta Bolognese contains:

Fat 0.5 g
Protein 3.5 g
Carbohydrates 27 g

We have the calories from the fat 0.5 x 9 = 4.5, from the protein 3.5 x 4 = 13, from the carbohydrates 27 x 4 = 108, so the total amount will be 4.5 + 13 + 108 = 125.5 calories. If we check the labels and make this kind of calculations, we can get our informations right away.

Task: Check your kitchen for different labels and look for the calories amount for a portion for at least three products.

And not we go back to misleading informations, as this is one of the challenges you need to overcome when you decide to eat healthier. Because even if it is not legal to lie about a food content, some producers will still try to misled you using a selective use of the information. Some of us, for example, will think that "Natural" means healthy. But it is not the case every time, as you can have meat or dairy, completely natural, but very high in fat. Or a natural fruit juice with a high content of sugar. Some labels will underline some of the natural ingredients and still have unhealthy additional content in the small print. It is only by reading the full content of a label that we are guarding ourselves from this kind of trickery.

Case study: Cereals for breakfast – Brand XYZ
Provides calcium, iron and vitamins.

Now, the package might contain vitamins and minerals, but the quantities are very small. And other ingredients in the cereals might be unhealthy, as for example the very high level of sugar.

Case study – Pre-prepared dinner – Brand XYZ
Reduced fat.

The amount of fat was reduced, but this does not means that the meal is automatically healthy. This particular food has originally contained 30 g of fats, and the new option has only 24 g of fat. The producer managed to reduce the fat by 20% and he can use this line in the product description, but with 24 g of fat, this meal is still high in fat. They can do the same thing for the salt or the sugar amount.

Case study – Breakfast cereals – Brand XYZ
Contains wholegrain rice.

You may think that this product is healthy, but the cereals are still very high in sugar. Also, it got a combination of wholegrain and processed wheat flour. There are many misleading words that can trigger a warning if we read them on any label, words like fresh, pure, light, low sugar, no added sugar, to quote just few of them.

***

Food additives – What are they and why are they used? Food additive are artificial or natural substances that are used in the manufacturing and processing of an ingredient, meal or drink to prolong shelf life, ad color, flavor or texture. Trying to make that food more appealing and safer. They can be natural, nature identical and artificial. Natural ones can be found in nature as a natural substance. They can be extracted from one food to be used in another. Like beetroot juice, that can be extracted from beetroot and used to give color for other foods. Nature identical are identically with the natural ones from the chemistry point of view, but are made by us, and they are used because they can be cheaper, stronger or more convenient and can be made in larger quantities. Artificial additives are made synthetically, and they are not copied after any natural substance. They are used to add color, flavor or sweeten. These additives can be found in brightly coloured sweets and diet or sugar free soft drinks. Some of them can be artificial and natural, depending on how they are produced. For example, the benzoic acid can be created synthetically and it is usually used in flavorings, jams, sweets, bakery, fizzy drink and ice cream. It is also found naturally in berries and prunes. It is a preservative , preventing bacteria and mold and the yeast for growing.

Why are these additives used and how many types exists?

The food producers use additives in food and drink for various reasons. Let's see what are them?

Antioxidants – their main quality is to prevent the food to turn rancid, due to the combination with the oxygen from the air. They are good for the food prepared with fat and oil, prolonging the shelf life. You can find antioxidants in meals like mayo, soups, pies, bakery products.

Colorants – are used when the food is losing its natural color due to cooking or processing, in order to make the food more attractive, by enhancing the colors and by giving a brighter appearance to the food. They are regulated and classified with a number, for example E150a is color caramel used for drinks like Coca Cola.

Emulsifiers – are usually added to help the ingredients to mix well together and to enable oil and water to be combined optimally.

Stabilizers and thickeners – are used to prevent the ingredients to separate once they are combined. The meal will increase viscosity (thickness) if we use a thickener and it can get a gel-like consistency if we use a gelling agent.

Preservatives – their main function is to prevent the growth of bacteria, fungus and mold, in order to maintain the food edible longer. There are traditional methods to preserve food using vinegar, salt or sugar. One of the most used preservatives is the benzoic acid. You can find them in jams, chutney, smoked fish, meat and cheese, cured meat and fish, processed food with long shelf life like canned and tinned ones.

Sweeteners – are added to food to make them to taste sweeter, are a substitution for natural sugar. They are used often to make diet versions of the soft drinks, to sweeten tea or coffee. Some sweeteners have the same level of sweetness like sugar (sorbitol), while others are much sweeter than sugar (saccharin).

Flavor enhancers – used to balance and enhance the flavors in a food product, without adding any new flavor. Salt is one of the most used ingredients to enhance taste, although it is not technically an additive, while monosodium glutamate is another, mostly used in ice cream, sweets like chocolate, biscuits, crisps or ready meals.

Task: Find some product with plenty of additives and see what you can find in the ingredients list. Bread, crisps, biscuits or ready meals are a good choice.

We often hear a lot of bad advertising related to the E numbers. What is that? Most of the people think that E is a code for artificial colors, but this is not the case. It is a term given to all the additives that are approved within the EU. Because they should be safe for people to eat, when put in the food, all the additives are tested and checked before they can be used in a product. Within the EU, they are evaluated by the European Food Safety Authority, and if they are safe and pass all the test, the additives are given an E number and added into a group according to their function. We have the following groups:
1. antioxidants (4-hexylresorcinol – E586, ascorbic acid – E300, tocopherols – E306),
2. colours (green S – E142, carotene – E160A, curcumin – E100),
3. emulsifiers (pectin – E440, lecithin – E322, invertase – E1103),
4. preservatives (benzoic acid – E210, sulphur dioxide – E220, sorbic acid – E200),
5. sweeteners (aspartame – E951, sorbitol – E420, sucralose – E955),
6. others (sodium citrates – E331, monosodium glutamate MSG – E622, citric acid – E330).

What are the advantages and disadvantages of the food additives?

The main advantages are regarding colour (more attractive meal colors, restoring food colors if lost or give color to colorless food), preservation (longer shelf life and less waste as the food doesn't need to be thrown away often), flavor (more appealing flavors or enhancers of the existing ones), texture (creating a desired viscosity or thickness or a gel like consistency, more effective binding for example for water and oil, ingredients will not separate once combined), added health benefits (fish oils like omega-3, vitamins and minerals can be added to the food, by boosting what is already present naturally or by artificially adding them).

The main disadvantages are regarding banned additives (it is up to each country to regulate the use of additives in the food products commercialized in that specific area), health risks (as additives are cheated in the laboratory, and short term and long term effects are unknown for many of them), allergies (especially children can be allergic or intolerant to some additives. If you have an eczema or asthma, it can worsen due to certain additives.), consumer knowledge (many do not know about the different additives used in food, as some products claim no artificial additives, yet they may still have naturally sourced additives in it).

We often hear negative stories about additives, but to what extent are they true? Can we find some positive examples too? You cannot test yourself for allergies, for example, for every additive that is in your food, potentially. It is not practical, neither safe. Having laws and regulations in place means that every new additive is tested and the consumers are informed about any possible danger. At the moment, UK follows the EU law related to the food additives. This law has very strict guidelines regarding the use of additives produced and sold in any country within the European Union. All the additives are testes for their purity and safety by the European Food Safety Agency – EFSA. If they are deemed safe to be eaten, they are given an E number and added to their list. The rules and standards set by the European Union are present in UK as The Food, Additives, Flavorings, Enzymes and Extraction Solvents (England) Regulations - 2013. The EU rules and standards are found in Regulation EC/1333/2008, setting up the rules on using food additives and the process needed for their use to be approved. These laws and regulations requires that additives are listed on the food labels, so we can make informed choices on what we eat and whether we want to consume certain additives. They also protect us from any harmful additive, by proving their benefits and side effects before they are approved.

***

There are some steps that you can use in order to create this habit of eating healthier and be happy with your diet. Let's talk about every one of these steps.

Step 1 – Start to use a food diary. You need to collect accurate data about your daily diet, in order to successfully create lasting change, at least for one week. You must record every time you eat what you eat and the amount of the meal.

Step 2 – Write about your ideal, individually tailored diet. Compare the plan with your existing diet. Once the analysis is done, you can proceed to the next step.

Step 3 – How we implement change, in order to follow a healthy diet.

Task: Can you tell me how healthy your diet is, from a scale from 1 to 10? (Tip: Keep your diary close to the place where you eat or prepare food, as in the kitchen or at the table in the dining room.)

About the healthy eating advice: what do we need to know? It is not only about how much you eat, but also about eating the right food, at the right time, in the right combination. A perfect diet will be balanced, following the right type, amount and variety of food.

Let's remind ourselves what we need.

Fruit and vegetables – minimum 33% or 5 portions. (Ideally fresh, but frozen or tinned also helps during winter time. Side note: potatoes are carbs, not veggies.)

Protein from meat or vegetarian sources – 15% or 2-3 portions.

Sugar and fat rich processed meals (for energy) – 1% meaning 1 portion or less.

Dairy (for calcium and protein) – 8% or 2-3 portions.

Carbohydrates (for energy, fibre, vitamins and minerals) – 33% of our diet.

How a healthy diet looks?

We need to include starchy foods such as bread, rice, potatoes, pasta, plenty of fruit and vegetables, enough milk and dairy foods and eggs and other non-dairy sources of protein (including nuts, tofu, beans, and pulses). Fatty and sugary foods are the last food group that you will eat. However, only a small amount of what you eat should be made up from fatty and sugary foods. Don't forget also to have plenty of fibre and a proper hydration. You may want to avoid to have saturated fat more than 10% of total fat intake, or to replace entirely the saturated fat with polisaturated fat. Eat at five to seven portions of fruit and vegetables per day. Eat some food that will provide Omega3 oil or use a natural supplement for it. Choose whole grains and nuts as snacks, have less than 6 g of salt daily. Avoid as much as possible: alcohol, processed meats or commercially produced foods (including 'ready meals') which tend to be high in salt and trans fatty acids, refined carbohydrates, such as white bread and processed cereals, sugar-sweetened drinks and high-calorie but nutritionally poor snacks, such as sweets, cakes and crisps.

Now we will become a bit specific with the advice, and we will tackle some issues that usually tend to appear. There are complex and simple carbohydrates. Complex ones are generally starchy foods like pasta, rice, potatoes, while simple ones are the sweet, full of sugar, foods. Ideally our diet needs to contain starchy, high in fibre carbs like wholemeal bread or cereals and brown rice. There is also the topic of the glycemic index, the rate of increase of the blood sugar level after a food is eaten. High glycemic index foods can lead to problems such as obesity and diabetes. High in fibre carbs as wholegrain cereals and brown rice will have a low glycemic index, being a healthier option to the processed, white bread, just to give one example. The latest researches will suggest seven portions of fruit and veg daily, instead of the well-known five-a-day, more veg than fruits, in order to provide the much needed fibre, preventing problems such as constipation or diverticular disease. They are also low in fat, make you to feel full, despite being low in calories and have most of minerals and vitamins. There are many tips and tricks to increase the proportion of fruit and veg in your diet:
-try some that you have not tried before, in different tastes and textures.
-add chopped apples, pears or bananas to your breakfast cereals.
-try to snack on fruits, and encourage your kids to do this also.
-use cherry tomatoes, dried fruits or carrot sticks as part of your lunch pack.
- include at least two or three vegetables with the main meals, steamed or stir fried.
-use fresh fruit juice instead of normal juice, buy a juice extractor or make it as a smoothie.
-have fruit based meals such as curries or stews with dried fruit, puddings or yogurt with fruit in it.
Talking about fibre, there are two kinds of them, soluble ones, found in oats, beans, peas and most of the fruit and veg, dissolving in water to form a gel-like substance, which increase the feeling of fullness and lower the cholesterol and sugar level in the blood, and the insoluble ones, found mostly in whole grains and fruit and veg skins, which cannot be digested, but helps with normal bowels movements.
Dairy is important as provider of protein and calcium, but some of it is also high in fat. Three servings a day are needed, low fat if it is possible. Non-dairy sources of calcium, such as leafy green veg, dried figs, almonds, sesame seeds and seaweed can be eaten if you avoid dairy, but you will need to add a source of vitamin D in order to enhance calcium absorption. You can find vitamin D in mushrooms or eggs, but most of it is generated by our skin combined with the sun rays. You need a decent amount of protein to keep yourself healthy, and not all of it can be provided by dairy. Meat is

not the ideal source of protein, although the majority prefers it. Fish is a bit better, providing also the essential fatty acids like omega-3. If you eat fish, try to increase the consummation of oily ones. Vegetables sources of proteins are not providing the right amount of amino acids and proteins if they are used alone, so you need to combine them with dairy and egg, if you are a vegetarian and avoid meat and fish. Your main meals must have two the following: grains, legumes or pulses, dairy products, eggs. Why I am talking about this? There is increasing evidence that eating meat (that has been processed in order to improve flavor or to preserve it longer) is linked with bowel, pancreas and prostate cancer, while it is also increasing the risk of stroke, heart diseases and type 2 diabetes. Related to fats, saturated ones from animal sources like meat are considered unhealthier than polyunsaturated ones, of vegetal origin. It is better to grill, bake or poach than to fry the food, cut or remove any excess fat from your meals, use low fat options where available, avoid cream, using yogurt instead. Learn your children to drink water of milk instead of sugary fizzy drinks, use fruits to add sweetness in meals, drink coffee or tea without sugar, do not eat too much chocolate or sweets, use herbs and spices instead of salt, for a different flavour, no added salt of the foods you buy is a good choice, avoid processed, fast food or takeaway, as they are high in salt. Even if you eat healthy, if you have bigger portions you will still gain weight, so try to use a smaller plate or eat as much as you need. Fill up of fruit and veg, and ask for a small portion when you are eating out. About drinking, water is containing zero calories, it is the best choice to hydrate, especially if you add a slice of lemon and keep it cool in the fridge. Milk is good too. Alcohol, in excess, can lead to liver, brain, pancreas and stomach problems, increasing your blood pressure, and adding weight as is containing too many calories. How can we calculate the right amount of alcohol? One unit of alcohol is 10 ml/8 g of pure alcohol, a half pint of beer, lager or cider, 25 ml of spirits or 50 ml of sherry or port. British Dietetic Association recommendations for men are the following: no more than 21 units weekly or 4 daily and at least 2 days a week to be alcohol free. Women should have less than 14 units weekly or 3 daily, and two alcohol free days a week. Pregnant women should not drink any alcohol. If you are vegetarian, you need to provide enough iron, B12 and omega-3 fatty acids. Good sources of iron include eggs, dried fruit, pulses, and dark green veg like broccoli, wholemeal bread and cereals. Good sources of vitamin B12 are eggs, milk, and cheese, yeast extracts like Marmite, breakfast cereals and soya products. Good sources of Omega-3 fatty acids for vegetarian are flaxseed and linseed oil, rapeseed oil, soy oil and soy based foods like tofu, eggs, walnuts. If you are vegan, that you need to provide yourself with enough calcium, vitamin D, B12, iron and Omega-3 fatty acids. For calcium and vitamin D you need unsweetened soy, rice and oats drinks, tofu, sesame seeds and tahini, pulses, brown bread, dried fruits. Exposure to sunlight will also increase your vitamin D levels. For iron you need to eat wholemeal bread and cereals, dark green leafy vegetables, nuts, dried fruits and pulses. For vitamin B12 you need to eat breakfast cereals, unsweetened soy drinks and yeast extract such as Marmite. For Omega-3 fatty acids you need to eat flaxseed, linseed or rapeseed oil, soy oil and soy based foods like tofu, walnuts.

Case study - Sheena

Sheena is a vegetarian, and she tries very hard to have varied meals. She has oats with a cup of milk for breakfast, baked potato, salad, soup or healthy sandwiches for lunch, but she likes to drink fizzy fruit juices, very sweet tea and snack on chocolate bars, crisps and sweets during her work. At dinner she usually cooks pasta, omelettes, and tofu or veggie burgers, followed by a cake or pudding.

Homework

Compare Sheena's diet with what you learn about healthy eating. This will also help you when you go to the next level and compare your own intake with what you learned.

____

____

____

Also, the takeaway and frozen meals often have high percentage of sugar, salt and fat, and when they are combined with decreasing the proportion of fruits and veggies in your diet, you will fail to provide the nutrients needed by the body. Let's see now if you can correctly identify which are the foods containing too much sugar, salt or fat.

Case study – Carly

Carly has cereals and a glass of fresh carrot or apple juice for breakfast. After that she will drink herbal tea or plain water. For lunch she will have salad with tuna, chicken or plain. For snack break, Carly will choose low fat rice cake, hummus, fruits or veg fingers. She like to eat out in the evening, and last week she had meaty pizza Monday, fish and chips Tuesday, spaghetti Bolognese Wednesday and chicken korma with rice, naan and mango chutney on Thursday.

Homework

Can you find any meal that may have a high percentage of sugar, salt or fat?

____

____

____

Your food diary needs to be accurate and effective. You need to write what it was consumed, at what time, amount and calories content of the meal, other additional information such as high content of sugar, salt or fibre. It is not difficult to keep a food diary. Take a look at our example.
Sheena's food diary entries for Friday - breakfast
Cereal – 50 g 140 kcal
Milk – 100 ml 50 kcal
Coffee with milk and 3 sugars – 1 cup 29 kcal -high in sugar
Quick view on Sheena's diet will make us to notice that she is eating the right amount of calories, she has all the needed fruits and veggies, her meals are balanced and she successfully substitute meat with black beans or other alternatives. On the bad side, she sometimes eats too many calories and she is having way too much sugar in her tea or as a snack (chocolate and biscuits). She can aim to eat more nuts, seeds and dairies.
If you are looking at your diet, what are the good and the wrong traits that you can identify?

____

____

____

You can take a look at the note you did at the start of your food diary. How accurate were you? Did you learn anything new that made you change your mind? Let's tick few lines related to your food diary. Use what you learn in the previous chapter to start to calculate how many calories you eat during an average day and how many calories you should eat. Check the five main food groups – carbohydrates, dairy, protein, fruits and vegetables, and how do you use this optimally. You already know about the 5 per day fruit and veg initiative. How are you dealing with this? Most adults should eat far less saturated fat, ideally less than 20 g per day. Same can be said about sugar, especially the hidden sugar from soft drink, sweets and even fast food meals. Salt must to be monitored too, no more than 6 g per day to be consumed. So, take a look at your diet now and try to find 10 ways to improve your diet.

CHAPTER 4
REACHING IDEAL WEIGHT

In this chapter we will start to learn about causes and symptoms of obesity, emaciation and malnutrition, risks linked to mentioned conditions, body mass index. After that we will speak about body image, feminine and masculine beauty, ideal body, pluses and minuses related to this and mass media influence to the matter. In the end of this chapter we will study how to have a balanced diet, why this is important, weight management, lifestyle and family and friends influence, truths and myths and, most important, how to make our own weight management program.

Ineffective weight management is usually a result of overeating or under eating, illness, inactive lifestyle or eating the wrong foods. Persisting in this erroneous ways will, in extreme cases, cause a medical condition which requires specialized assistance. The main problems related to wrong weight management are emaciation, malnourishment and obesity.

Emaciation is medical condition present in the less developed countries, where is not enough food and it is hard for children, elderly and people with disabilities to feed themselves properly. They will look thin, as they are not eating enough because of their lifestyle, health problems or circumstances. The body is not having the daily amount of nutrients, beginning to burn fat and muscle for energy, resulting in rapid weight loss. This happens when you are not eating enough or you are eating the wrong type of food. Other cause of emaciation can be an existing health issue that is preventing the body to absorb the required nutrients. The main symptoms are frailness and dramatic weight loss, but you can also notice extreme fatigue, passive behavior, depression, excessively dry mouth, severe dehydration, circulatory problems and improper organs function.

Malnutrition happens when the body is not getting the right amount of nutrients. It is also named malnourishment, which translate as poor nutrition. Can be caused by an inadequate amount of nutrients in somebody diet or as a result of an illness making the body to not absorb the nutrients from the food properly. Extreme malnourishment is a common sight in countries where access to food is difficult or impossible. Low income or long term health conditions can also make it difficult for some to get the right amount of nutrients. The symptoms associated with malnutrition are sudden weight loss, depression, constant fatigue and immunity level decrease.

Obesity is characterized by a person who is dramatically overweight, carrying a large amount of body fat. It is a growing problem in the fast developing countries, as a result of inactive lifestyle combined with unhealthy diet. Eating a lot of fatty foods such as takeaways and pre-packed meals, large portions, drinking a lot of alcohol and living a sedentary life will put you at risk of becoming obese. Obesity symptoms are fatigue, increased sweating, sleeping difficulty, back or joints pain and breathlessness.

In order to determine whether somebody is or not at their ideal weight, the health professionals use a number known as body mass index or BMI. You can easily find a BMI tool online to check your own index.

When we are thinking at emaciation, we associate this with the images of severely emaciated children in the developing world. However, this is a global problem, happening for a number of different reasons, most of the cases because the body is not receiving the right amount of vitamins and minerals. This will result in frailty and rapid weight loss. Hunger and starvation are associated with poverty, due to the lack of availability of food with the required nutrients, people being unable to afford the adequate food to maintain themselves healthy. Elderly and people with disability may also struggle to maintain a healthy and sustainable diet. A severe illness can make it difficult to consume the correct nutrients, especially if the subject is bedridden. Other pre-existing health conditions can decrease our body's ability to absorb nutrients, leading to weight loss. Diabetes type 1, for example, can prevent the body to produce the energy required for daily use, causing dramatic weight loss and even emaciation, in more than few occasions. Anorexia and bulimia, to quote just few of the main eating disorders, have become a prevalent issue in the developed countries. This kind of eating disorders will often result in sudden weight loss and additional health issues. Bulimics can experience teeth and throat damage due to vomiting and stomach damage while anorexics may suffer of hearth problems, damaged livers and kidneys because they do not eat enough food.

We would say that someone is emaciated when they are not eating enough or fail to provide the required nutrients in order to maintain their body healthy. I will write now about the health risks associated with emaciation. Anemia, when an individual has a lower number or red blood cells than normal, is often present at the people who are underweight, because they fail to eat a balanced diet providing them with essential iron. This will cause breathlessness, tiredness and chest pains. If you are underweight, you are also at risk to become infertile. Emaciation, for men, will affect the body's ability to produce healthy sperm because of the lack of the required vitamins and minerals while women can have ovulation and menstruation problems that will make it difficult to become pregnant.

Emaciation impair the body ability to recognize when it needs water, resulting in dry skin and dehydration, combined with lack of nutrients this can disturb the activity of liver and kidneys, ultimately resulting in organ failure. Lack of essential vitamins and minerals can induce a deficiency of the immune system, often starting a chain reaction. For example the lack of vitamin D can affect the ability to metabolize calcium, weakening the bones and joints, while vitamin C insufficiency can cause weakness and fatigue. If you are underweight, you are also at risk of osteoporosis, a disease that causes the bones to become fragile and break easily, making fractures more likely. This is usually a result of vitamin D and calcium deficiency, combined with lack of exercise.

It is a sign of malnutrition if a person is significantly under the ideal weight. Using BMI, you can determine right away if somebody it at risk. A BMI between 18.5 and 20 is at risk of malnourishment, a BMI under 18.5 may be considered at a high risk. But emaciation and sudden weight loss are not the only indicators of malnutrition. Even if you are healthy or overweight, you can still be malnourished if you are not eating the right food. The main symptoms are: weight loss, gradually or sudden, depression, slower recovery from other illnesses, diarrhea, lack of focus, slow healing wounds, irritability.

Another big concern is about being overweight, as this can have a considerable impact on your health. Obesity is lowering the life expectancy for both men and women, added to many short term and long term health issues. Some researchers put obesity in the same category with cancer, high blood pressure and diabetes, thinking about the detrimental effect on someone's health. It is also directly linked to depression and low self-esteem, this making it difficult for an overweight person to lose weight through diet and lifestyle changes. We are talking now about what the today's media refer as "obesity crisis", and the cost of tackling this problem is enormous. In United Kingdom alone, one of every seven children is clinically obese. We are blaming things like Xbox, computers and tablets, but the reality is that the real issue is the lack of knowledge about a balanced diet and the chronic inactivity. Let's see what are the main issues linked to obesity. If you are pregnant and overweight, there is an increased risk of miscarriage and potentially problems for mother or child. It could be hard for clinically obese to make positive changes in their lifestyle and diet.

Case study

Daniel and his struggle with weight

Daniel is in his twenties and he was overweight for as long as he remembers. He find it difficult to buy clothes that fit, was often bullied in school, and he rarely goes anyway except to work, because he thinks he is not good at socializing with colleagues and has low self-esteem. He is aware that he must lose weight, and he asked his doctor for advice about eating healthy and exercising, but it is difficult for him to commit to lasting changes in his diet and lifestyle.

Karen and the lack of exercise

Karen is 43 and she is a career woman working in a top position in her company. She used to be fit and active in her youth, but now most of the time she is solving high pressure tasks related to her job. She doesn't have always time to cook, and very often she will just order some food (usually containing a lot of salt and fat).

Obesity can influence one's quality of life, creating a vicious circle, because the more you eat, you become inactive, and you have time to eat more and so on.

Task: Think at 10 possible advices for our case study.

1. ____
2. ____
3. ____
4. ____
5. ____
6. ____
7. ____
8. ____
9. ____
10. ____

Next on the list is the subject of the body image and how this is influenced by media. I am too tall! Too thin! Too fat! Too short! You will say, under the invisible pressure of the overwhelming presence of the modern ideals of beauty. Depending on their mindset, people can have a positive or a negative body image, and serious conditions such as eating disorders can result because of the way some people see themselves, as opposed as how they really are. We form an idea of our body image by comparing it with friends, people we know or celebrities from the mass-media. If it is something that we do not like, we will start to accept a negative comparison related to our body. The way you react at other people perception of yourself can impact and decide if you will create a negative or a positive body image. It is all about focus, as a person focused on negatives can easily ignore all the compliments and good things people said about her/him. The other way, ignoring the negative things said by others and accepting only the positives seems to work better in terms of self-esteem and positive body image, as long as you are not becoming unreachable, forming a much better opinion about yourself than you are in reality. The best way is the middle way, knowing exactly your value, your best and least developed qualities, because if you learn more about yourself, the other's opinion will not affect you. At the end of the day, your body image is just an image reflecting what you believe is the reality, but not the reality itself. The ideal of beauty is changing from one period to another, anyway, and what is considered beautiful today could not be the same with what the next generation will accept as a truth. In Renaissance, for example, we can see that the ideal body image for a woman was a full-figured body, as more fat suggested more wealth and affluence. A full-figured body was the norm until the 19th century, when the corset was invented, women wanting to underline their hips. The idea evolved, but it was only at the beginning of the 20th century when the idea of a slender woman becomes attractive. Starting from that period, the ideal feminine body changed, and a slighter body shape was desired. But, it was not until 1980, when diet and weight loss become a successful business. This continues 20 years later, moving even further from reality, due to the computer and the paint brushing programs, which can manipulate photos of the actresses and models, giving them unrealistic body proportions and flawless complexions. As for the masculine body, an athletic, muscular body shape was desired from as far back as the ancient Rome and Greece. Renaissance painters worshiped tall and muscular men, and everything was alright until 1950, when impossibly muscular physique was promoted. Everyone started to want to look like elite male athletes, without realizing they spend their whole life staying fit, through rigorous training and diet. The 21st century culture also emphasized on personal hygiene and professional grooming. In our times, the modern man should be incredibly physically fit, in perfect health, with perfect hair, flawless skin and no unsightly hair on his body. But while the human male body may not have undergone under such a drastic change like the female body, there is an increasing pressure in our actual culture related on how we need to look, placing some unrealistic expectations on any normal individual.

The body image is a tricky concept to deal with, as we often refer to our ideal body, a product of the modern society, media and western culture, in our case, promoted by fashion models and movie stars. This ideal is unrealistic, a product of a life of training and restrictions made by professionals paid for the ideal of a perfect body. Accepting that your body is different than the ideal one is the first step to a positive body image while being upset because you notice the difference will lead to a negative body image. If you cultivate a positive body image, you will be comfortable with your appearance and feel little to no anxiety or stress watching yourself in the mirror. You are not looking to match the ideal promoted by the society, and you know that your self-worth is not linked mostly on how you look. If you build a negative body image, you will not have a realistic perception of yourself, and that version of yourself in your mind will not match the one from the mirror. You need to stop comparing yourself with others very often and realize that your family, friends and society will not expect you to reach that ideal body shape.

Here are few tips about how to maintain a positive body image. Try to pay compliments to yourself and avoid self-criticism. Focus on those aspects of your appearance that you can change. Do not even think about what you cannot change. Always keep in mind what is unique and interesting about you. Aim for and maintain a healthy and strong body.

Task: Find five ways of thinking for a person with negative body image. Do the same for one with positive body image. Which are the differences?

In the modern times we are exposed to an endless stream of images of what they believe is the perfect human body. We have television, smartphones, movies and magazines, and it is difficult for someone to escape from all the subtle suggestions that our media is promoting.

Case study – Brenda

7.15 Brenda is awake and is checking the latest news on her phone. On the side we can see an ad for a new range of jewels featuring a smartly dressed couple – wife and husband.
8.00 She will have Weetabix and hot milk for breakfast. On the cereals box is a woman in bikini, with a toned body, advising to use that brand of cereals.
8.45 Few minutes until she is leaving for work, Brenda turns the TV on to check the weather, presented by a slender weather girl, with a beautiful

make-up.

9.00 On the bus to work, hers is decorated with ads for a new gym that has just opened on her street, with a physique of a muscular man.

11.00 While having their breakfast, Brenda and her colleagues talk about a TV show where the presenters are discussing about the dresses worn by celebrities at the previous night movie award ceremony.

13.00 During her lunch, she is looking in a magazine, reading and article about a singer who put on some weight. There are also other articles with glamorous pictures of other pop singers and TV stars.

18.00 The work finished, Brenda will go to cinema with friends to see the latest movie played by the same actresses she'd read about when she had lunch.

22.00 Once she is at home, she will take a look in a lingerie catalogue featuring slim, toned models using the available products.

Task: Can you find and underline all the ways that Brenda has been exposed during one of her normal work day?

____
____
____

____

We are talking here about internet ads, food packaging, TV shows, billboards, celebrities, movies, magazines and product catalogues. There are two sides here, talking about media and the effects of this constant exposure to advertising. There are some suggesting that all this will influence women and men to have unrealistic expectations about their body image, resulting in trying dangerous diets and increasing the eating disorders. Others think that the friends and family have a greater influence on one's expectations of his/her physical appearance, and that media can help with weight management advice. And this is partially true, as individuals growing up in supportive families tend to have a positive body image, while women constantly exposed to images of skinny models and photoshoped images can sometimes set unrealistic targets for personal weight. Being constantly bombarded with images of fit, healthy men can inspire some to eat healthier and exercise more, but in the Western society where being skinny is the norm, the number of people suffering from eating disorders increased in the last years. However, there is a recent trend to appreciate real beauty, to promote more natural body shapes and diversity. But this is not yet the norm of every television or celebrity magazine.

Task: During one day, observe yourself and see how many times you find being influenced by the ideal body image advertised around you.

Case study - Stanley

When Stanley was young, he was very active, ate balanced meals and was always in the right place on the BMI scale. But, as he get older, he tried to achieve that lean, muscular body promoted by his favorite movie star, using supplements for muscle mass and going to gym Monday to Friday. He start to find it difficult to maintain his healthy weight and his BMI fluctuates when he stop doing exercise.

Case study – Adrian

Adrian developed an obsession about her weight; always thinking what kind of food she needs to buy and which is the next designer diet. Looking at her BMI, she is a bit overweight, but she has a healthy diet and lifestyle. Despite this, she was often unhappy with her body image and self-conscious when comparing with the TV stars. It was a series of TV shows on the local channel, promoting normal, fully shaped woman that made her more comfortable with her own physique and prone to decrease her regular dieting attempts.

Next, we will learn more about effective methods of weight management, the role of a balanced diet, what are the implications of the energy balance, how the lifestyle choices impact on weight management, and the most common weight loss myths.

Eating a moderate amount is not everything, as you need to get the right nutrients in the right amount, if you want to stay healthy and have the correct weight. The food you ate is directly related to your weight, let's check the main food groups as a reminder. Starchy foods such as potatoes, pasta, rice or bread should be 33% of your diet. Protein rich foods like eggs, beans or any other source must be eaten up to three portion daily. Fruits and vegetables are also needed for fibre and most of the vitamins and minerals. Dairy (milk, yogurt, cheese) is another important source of protein. High fat or sugary products provide only a short energy boost, and should be avoid if is not a necessity. Too much fat, salt of sugar can lead to an increase of what you eat daily, causing weight gain. Some other key nutrients missing from your diet can lead to weight loss and not enough energy for your daily tasks. A balanced diet is important to maintain a healthy weight, and variety is the key. In UK, what you call a normal diet is usually very high in fat, salt and sugar, creating health risk such as high blood pressure, heart disease or diabetes.

You remember how you learn in Chapter 1 about BMR (basal metabolic rates) and how this is linked with your body's energy needs. The basal metabolic rate is the rate of the energy used by a person for the basic functions of the body. Add the energy needed for the exercise and movement and the result is equal with the total energy requirement for one person per day. The first rule of the weight management is to aim to have a calorie intake equal or lower than the total energy requirement. To say it in plain language, the calorie intake is the energy going in and the energy requirement is the energy coming out of our body. Let's see some examples.

Case study – Gabriel

Calories intake is equal with the energy requirement.

Gabriel eats a healthy and balanced diet and gets 2100 calories daily. Using a BMR calculator, he found that he has a BMR of 1800. He also goes to gym and burns 300 calories per training.
Energy in: 2100
Energy out: 1800+300=2100

Gabriel's weight will stay the same.

Case study – Angel

Calories intake is bigger than the energy requirement.

Angel is eating healthy and balanced meals, but she like to snack on sweets and occasionally she will drink a can of Coke. On average, she has a calories intake of 2300 calories. Her BMR is 1750, but she is running 1-2 miles every day, burning 250 calories.
Energy in: 2300
Energy out: 1750+250=2000

Angel's weight will increase over time.

Case study – Sheldon

Calories intake is lower than the energy requirement.

Sheldon is a professional athlete doing interval running and high intensity training, burning on average 480 calories every day. His BMR is 1600, so his total energy requirement is 2080 calories per day. He is very cautious and is eating only vegetarian food, managing to provide all the key nutrients. His calories intake is 1800 per day.

Energy in: 1800

Energy out: 1600+480=2080

Sheldon's weight will decrease over time.

Our energy requirement is not the same every day, and the previous examples are right only if we can see them as a habit, day to day basis. You will not get fat just because one day you will eat only fast food, and you will not get slim just because you eat salad only two days a week. Of course, this can help, but it is not enough. Your average energy requirements needs to be positive of negative for weeks or months, in order to gain or lose weight. Learning about your energy requirements and adjust it according to your needs is just the first step in achieving your ideal weight. You need to know what to change, to implement it and maintain it over a longer period of time to achieve considerable results. I will tell you few well known tips about weight management. If you are underweight, increase your calorie intake, decrease the level of exercises and avoid food and drink high in fat and sugar, as those have a direct link to body fat, not to body mass. If you have a healthy weight level, maintain the same calorie intake, do moderate exercises and do not eat high fat or high sugar food or drinks in excess. If you are overweight, increase your physical activity level, decrease your level of calorie intake and avoid at all costs high sugar or high fat meals.

Case study

Natalie and Steven weight close to 180 pounds and they want to lose 10 pounds over the next 10 weeks. They did the checks and found out the goal is achievable if the reduce their daily energy requirements with 150 calories.

In order to work out the details, the "energy input" must be 150 calories less than the "energy output". Natalie is working most of the time, so she decide to eat less, while Steven has the extra time to increase the exercise amount. To achieve her goal, Natalie can drink water instead of Coke, eat salad at lunch instead of chips, use tuna fish canned in water instead of oil. To achieve his goal, Steven can go to gym for 30 minutes, do a half an hour bike ride, run one mile or play football for 20 minutes.

Task: Can you think to 4 different approaches for Natalie and Steven to achieve their objectives?

____

____

____

____

____

One thing is clear when we are talking about weight management. To achieve your perfectly balanced weight is a matter of lifestyle, not a quick fix. You do not need to become obsessed, or to follow draconic diets, only to do the right choices 90% of the time. You can have the occasional drink or even 2 slices of cheesecake, as long as this is not a daily occurrence. Crash diets and endless gym sessions will work on the short term but, as you are using will as motivation, and not the process of creating a habit, you will stop eventually and sooner or later you will revert to the original condition. What are the main diets hacks to help you to achieve this perfect physical balance? Snacking can bring you down or take you up, depending on how you do it. If you are having fruits and nuts for a snack, this is a good habit to provide you the extra energy needed to perform optimally in a stressful day. But if chocolate and crisps are your main type of snacks, this is a bad habit, and bringing all hat extra sugar and fat will make it difficult for you to lose weight. Sleep is another effective tool in your fight with the extra weight, and a good night sleep is required, a continuously 8-9 hours program, ideally going to bed early and waking up early will do the trick. Too much or too little rest will impact your body negatively, resulting in activity spikes, less energy, fatigue and lack of motivation in doing exercises. Fast food is not always a good choice, but as I said, if you are eating high quality, nutrient rich, organic food most of the times, then you can have something that you enjoy occasionally. Alcohol and smoking are a bad combination, as a pint of lager will have 180 "empty" calories, and nicotine is acting like an appetite suppressant, while difficulties with breathing make you more likely to decrease your physical activity. The closest circle of friends and family, if they have developed bad habits as drinking, smoking and ordering fast food often, will make it hard for us to maintain healthy habits.

Case study

Angelina

Angelina was working for the last seven years for a major charity. She enjoys her work, but lately she has noticed that her health is not what used to be, due to the fact that sometimes she is working extra hours and eating unhealthy sugary snacks for a short time energy boost. For the same reasons, she will not follow a proper sleeping schedule, and this will decrease her motivation for exercise.

Bruce

Bruce's parents and grandparents planned their meals in advance and bought only fresh, organic, healthy food. They weren't eating ready meals or takeaways more than few times per year, both parents cooking from scratch, with fresh ingredients. Now, when Bruce has a family on his own, he rarely eat takeaways, cooking with his wife and providing a balanced, home-cooked diet, such as the one he ate as a child.

Liam and Annabelle

Liam and Annabelle are friends, and they got a lot of other neighbors and colleagues to invite them out for a drink or a meal, at least 3-4 nights a week. Annabelle is not drinking alcohol usually, but sometimes her peers pressure her into drinking more. She is trying to lose weight, but her nights out will make her gym session next day difficult to attend. Liam is always on the run, having two jobs and not enough time, and he like to prepare a ready meal fast and eat it on his breaks. But after he went with some of his friends to a yoga retreat holiday, and he ate only vegetarian, organic, fresh food, he was surprised how the taste is much better and his energy increased. Soon after coming back, Liam started to learn how to cook his own food at home.

Task: Do a summary of your own eating habits and see if you can find at last three ways to increase your health and improve your own weight management.

____
____
____
____
____.

In the next paragraph we will introduce you to some of the most commons weight loss myths and see why they aren't true.

Myth #1
You need to starve yourself in order to lose weight.

What we know today as crash dieting, or extreme dieting, is one of the common errors which an uninitiated person can do, on the same level with extra exercise regime. The problem is that, while you are not provided with the most needed nutrients, you are more prone to fall for high sugar or high fat for to compensate the lack of energy, sabotaging yourself on the long term.

Myth #2
Fast weight lose can be achieved with a long, strenuous physical training.

You can do this for a limited time, and you can even lose significant weight, but, because you are using sheer force of will instead of building healthy habits, you will come back to your normal diet and stop exercising after a while, getting your lost weight back very fast. The best way to do it is by decreasing your calorie intake moderately and exercising 3-4 days a week. 15 minutes high intensity training, for example, can burn the same amount of calories as a 90 minutes unmotivated training at the gym. Training with moderation and decreasing our calorie intake with a minimal percentage will help us to get better results on the long term.

Myth #3
It is good to lose weight when your main strategy is to skip main meals.

Definitely not. Skipping meals will only make you to snack more often on food high in sugar or fat, in order to get the much needed energy, you will not provide to your body the right amount of nutrients and you will get tired much faster. As you learned already, the best way to do this is by reducing your calories intake gradually with a small percentage, while you increase your calories burned doing exercises.

Myth #4
You will put on weight if you eat too many carbohydrates.

You are not using carbs only for weight, but also as main source of energy. They are also rich in starch, and starch should make 33% of your diet. They are good carbs, such as brown rice and whole grains, and bad carbs, such as white bread. The problem is that even wholemeal bread is lately containing a lot of chemicals and additives. Read the label to find out more about what you eat every day.

Myth #5
If you cut out all your snacks, you can lose weight faster.

The snacks are not the problem, but what we consider as being snacks it is important, as we are eating snacks in order to boost our energy thorough the day. Snacks such as nuts, vegetables and fruits are always welcome, while crisps and chocolate bars are not such a good idea.

Myth #6
Eating a healthy diet is very expensive.

This one it is simply not true. It is much cheaper to cook from scratch than to buy ready frozen meals, and if we are talking about snacks, an apple or an orange is cheaper that a chocolate bar or a packet of crisps. Also, cooking from scratch, you can easily make more than one portion and save it to eat it later.

Myth #7
It is very easy and effortless to achieve weight loss using slimming pills.

Slimming pills can help if they are used while you maintain a balanced, healthy diet and active lifestyle habits. But trying to use only the pills to magically get your ideal weight will never work.

Myth #8
Margarine has a lower fat content than butter.

Butter has more saturated fat than margarine, but it is likely to contain less hydrogenated fat. When you are trying to maintain a healthy lifestyle, thinking in terms of fat content, both saturated and hydrogenated fats are equally bad when they are in excess.

Myth #9
Products with reduced fats or reduced sugar content are very healthy.

If a product is marked as 'reduced fat' or 'reduced sugar', they will have less fat or sugar than the full fat or full sugary products, but it can be still high in fat or sugar, and containing a lot of salt and many additives.

Myth #10

You can lose weight fast if you are drinking water.

Drinking the right amount of water every day is important to stay fit and healthy, however it will not impact on your weight, as the water calorie intake is 0 (zero). Skipping meals and drinking water instead can lead to an increase in snacks, often unhealthy ones.

These are the most commons myths about weight loss. Once we become familiar with it, we can reach the next level, creating a weight management program. There are many examples, and we can use one that was already tested around the world, or we can make our own weight management program. What is the logical sequence in making your own?

What is my current weight? What is my desired weight? What is my ideal weight? Check what is your basal metabolic rate – BMR, and your personal activity level. Add them together to find your daily calorie consumption. Then decide the time interval to achieve the desired weight (which is better to be close to your ideal weight, or you need to read again about the biases of the self-image). Whatever is your time interval, my advice is to set the double of it as the time to achieve your goal. Now set some intermediary periods and achieve the secondary goals. Like if you want to lose 6 pounds in 3 months, the intermediary goal is to lose 2 pounds every month. Your secondary goals need to be challenging, but achievable. There is a rule called the 3M rule, which can help you to remember how to set a weight management program. They are milestones, monitoring, maintaining.
1. Milestones – secondary goals on your way to the final goal.
2. Monitoring – to achieve every milestone or adjust your strategy if you miss one of it.
3. Maintaining – the strategy used after you achieve your goal.

Case study – Riley

Riley currently weights 86 kg. She would like to lose 12 kg using a combination of diet, interval running and high intensity training, and she plan to do this in 4 months.

Riley journal - milestones

Week 1
One half an hour running session.
Snack only one raw chocolate bar instead of two normal chocolate bars.
Weight to achieve: 86 kg

Week 2
Two half an hour running sessions.
Add one fruit and one veg portion to daily meals
Weight to achieve: 85.5 kg

Week 3
Two half an hour running sessions.
Walking to work instead of bus – 4 miles one return trip.
Takeaway once per week only.
Weight to achieve: 85 kg

Week 4
Three half an hour running sessions.
Bowl of raisins and nuts instead of crisps for snacking.
Weight to achieve: 84 kg

Week 5
Three half an hour running sessions.
One salad and one extra fruit for snack daily.
Weight to achieve: 83.5 kg

Week 6
One half an hour swimming session at the local pool.
Three running sessions – two interval running and one 5k run.
Weight to achieve: 82.5 kg

Week 7
Eat 5-per-day fruits every single day.
Three running sessions – two interval running and one 5k run.
Weight to achieve: 82 kg

Week 8
Have only fruits and nuts instead of sugary or fatty snacks.
Three running sessions – one interval running and two 5k runs
Weight to achieve: 81 kg

Week 9
Have a salad and at least one other meal made from scratch.
Two half an hour swimming sessions at the local pool.
Three interval running sessions, at least 30 minutes each.
Weight to achieve: 80 kg

Week 10

Healthy snacks only.
Three daily meals made from scratch every day when possible.
Three half an hour swimming sessions at the local pool.
Two 5k runs.
Weight to achieve: 79 kg

Week 11
One swimming session 1 hour long.
Three 5k runs.
Fresh cooked meals made from scratch every day.
Weight to achieve: 78 kg

Week 12
One continuous 15k run
Two 30 minutes swimming sessions.
5-per-day every day.
Weight to achieve: 77 kg

Week 13
Cooking from scratch with fresh ingredients.
Two one-hour long swimming sessions.
Two 5k runs.
Weight to achieve: 76 kg

Week 14
At least 70% of my diet to be water rich foods.
Two one-hour long swimming sessions with 0.5 ankle weight.
Two 5k runs.
Weight to achieve: 75 kg

Week 15
At least 70% of my diet to be alkaline.
Two one-hour long swimming sessions with 0.5 ankle weight.
One 10k run, one 5k run.
Weight to achieve 74.5 kg

Week 16
Maintaining the 70% water rich, 70% alkaline diet.
Two 20 minutes continuous swimming.
Two 10k runs.
Weight to achieve: 74 kg.

Task: Draft your own weight management program. Check your own weight and see if you need to lose or gain weight, establish and interval to achieve your perfect weight and think about what changes you need to make in your diet and exercise regimen in order to achieve your goal.

You will probably need to follow the next steps. What are your goals for the weight management program? I want to reach 77 kg and 15% body fat after 7 months. What is the information available to start your plan? At the present moment, my weight is 84 kg and my body fat is 24.6%.

What I need to know about setting up a short term weight management program? Setting a realistic goal is the most important part, from the point of view related to motivation and success. If your goal is unrealistic, you are more likely to give up, lose motivation and stop at some moment before the proposed term.
Case study
Gabriel and Michael

Gabriel and Michael want to achieve the optimal weight, losing few pounds, so they decide to set up a weight management program. How can you do it properly? Michael will use the SMART method, while Gabriel is not so technical.

Specific target weight
Gabriel – want to lose a bit of weight.
Michael – want to lose 7.5 kg.

Measurement
Gabriel – will check himself in the mirror to see the progress.
Michael – will check his weight daily to see when he will lose all the 7.5 extra kilograms

Attainable goal
Gabriel – is thinking that will probably fail. No timeline set.
Michael – checked on internet health websites and with his GP to be sure that the weight is ideal and the timeline is good.

Relevance
Gabriel – is doing this only because his friend Michael is doing it.
Michael – want to lose weight for his wedding in 4 months from now, as he needs to fit in his brand new tuxedo.

Timeline

Gabriel – has no starting date or finishing date. He hopes to do it in few months.

Michael - has a weekly goal for the next 4 months, and he will finish it on 4th of August.

Task: If you were Michael, can you think at some ways to help Gabriel to achieve   his   goal?

____

____

____

____

____

Key points

Now is the time to prepare a weight gain/loss/maintaining program for you. Try to use the SMART method. You may also apply what you just learned about final goal, timescale, tracking progress and milestones. When you start, collecting all the information needed is a must. But before that, knowing what information is needed and why will improve your chances of being successful. Read the study cases explained before. Take notes if you like to do it. Once you collected all the information needed, it is the right time to start planning your weight management program.

Here is how you start

Month 1 goals

Running 3 times a week, at least 1 mile.
Doing a strength training once a week
Doing one yoga session daily
Doing 5 minutes of martial art training
Coca Cola once per week only.
Sugary sweets twice per week only

Month 1 milestones check

Kg 84 =>83
Body fat 24%=>22%

Here are few tips for every kind of weight management program.

If you want to lose weight, aim for a daily calorie intake reduction of at least 500 kcal. Do not try to lose more than 1 kg per week, as this is an example of unhealthy diet. To lose 1 kg of fat, you need to burn 7000 kcal.

If you want to maintain your actual weight, you can do more exercise when you feel like eating a bit extra, you still need to avoid foods that are high in fat or high in sugar and try to eat different kind of food with a similar nutrient content, for variation.

If gaining weight is your goal, you should chose food that is rich in nutrients, such as nuts, dried fruits or bee honey. Aim to increase your calories intake by 600-1000 daily. Keep in mind that you need a 7000 extra calories to gain one extra kg.

CHAPTER 5
EATING DISORDERS

In this chapter we will define the term "eating disorder" and we will describe all the possible types of eating disorder. We already know that everyone had a different eating habit, which can be influenced by a number of factors. We cannot define precisely how a normal eating habit looks, but we can identify quite accurate what a disturbed or abnormal eating habit looks, and that is usually called eating disorder.

It is all starting in the mind, when one is judging himself too harsh and is obsessively thinking about putting on weight. That person will be very conscious about what he is eating, finding ways to restrict his calories intake, due to a faulty self-image. But an eating disorder is not only about losing weight. It could be a disturbed eating habit that is including over eating too. If you think about, one person can be healthy, with normal weight or overweight. In UK only, more than one and a half million people are suspected of having an eating disorder. Women are the main majority, approx. 90%, but men numbers are increasing lately. There are three main eating disorders: anorexia nervosa, bulimia nervosa and binge eating disorder (BED).

Having an eating disorder can have disastrous consequences on your health, but you should always be diagnosed by a specialist. The doctors will often use what is called SCOFF test, to underline the signs of any eating disorder. The following questions are asked:

-Do you ever make yourself sick because you ate too much?
-Do you ever worry that you are out of control about how much you eat?
-Do you recently lost more than 10 kg or more than one stone?
-Do you think that you are fat, even if other people say that you are thin?
-Is food having control over your life?

When it is not one of the three main eating disorders, the specialist is mentioning the diagnosis of Eating Disorder Not Otherwise Specified (EDNOS). This is the name used in the Diagnostic and Statistical Manual of Mental Disorders (DSM) classification system up to and including 2013. If one's symptoms were not the ones of anorexia or bulimia, or they were a mix of both, there were identified as EDNOS. This term stopped to be used lately.

The most known eating disorder is Anorexia Nervosa, and this is noticed often and sanctioned in mass media, due to the severe nature of its physical effects. About 20% of the people having Anorexia die because of it, making it the illness with the highest rate of death of all psychological illnesses. Despite this, Anorexia is the least common eating disorder, in UK for example, only 10% of eating disorder sufferers are anorexic. Anorexia can have short-term and long-term effects on someone health. In the short-term, the anorexic person becomes emaciated, look malnourished, has poor skin and hair, is dehydrated, feeling weak and tired, can present depression, sadness and low self-esteem, the facial hair increases, fine hair start to grow on the body. In the long-term, the anorexic person will become anemic, will present irregular heartbeat, chance to heart disease, kidney damage and failure, osteoporosis and difficulty in getting pregnant or dangerous pregnancy is increased. They are prone to fits and seizures, low blood sugar and low blood pressure. Sometimes brittle bones or loss of menstrual periods is also encountered. Both short and long-term symptoms can have a significant impact on a person health, very fast. Psychological effects on the partners and families of someone suffering from Anorexia were also noted.

One of the most encountered eating disorder is Bulimia Nervosa, accounted for 40% of the people suffering from eating disorder in UK. These are an illness characterized by cycles of eating large amounts of food and get it out through laxatives or vomiting (bingeing and purging). The effects on short-term are dehydration, abdominal pain, bloating, tooth decay, chronic sore throat and mouth sores induced by vomiting, in case of using laxatives we can observe constipation and problems with the bowels, the fine blood vessels from the inside of the eyes can break, general weakness and dizziness, swelling of the hands, feet and salivary glands, puffy cheeks. In the long-term effects we mention ruptured stomach or esophagus, low potassium levels, low blood pressure and low sugar, fits, seizures, kidney damage and failure, irregular heartbeats, heart disease, anemia, osteoporosis, loss of menstruation for females. Bulimia by itself can be life threatening, with side effects affecting the person's life and health for long time, even after recovery.

qBinge eating disorder (also known as BED) is found to every second person suffering from an eating disorder (50% of the people), but it is not a well-known eating disorder, receiving less attention from the mass-media. BED main behavior is involving compulsive over-eating. Some people suffering from this disorder are dieting and over-eating as a habit, so it is not always easy to spot it on. The short-term effects are constipation or diarrhea, consistent sugar cravings, headaches and tremors due to the blood sugar levels, obesity, hair and skin problems, anxiety, depression, and physical discomfort after over-eating, unhappiness, and low self-esteem. The long-term effects such as asthma, sleep apnea, diabetes type 2, cancer, heart disease, high cholesterol, kidney and liver failure, strokes, back pain, gastro-esophageal reflux, high blood pressure, infertility.

Case study - Lauren

Lauren works the whole day, she intent to cook when she come home, but she find herself in front of the TV watching her favorite soap-drama, with some biscuits and few packs of crisps. But this is only the beginning, and she will raid the cupboards later, looking for something sweet. Lauren is obese, and sometimes she decides to diet and eat healthier, only for a couple of days, the binges kicking back even stronger. She knows she is over-eating, she blame her lack of will for that, but she cannot stop to have some chocolate biscuits if they are offered to her. The main effect of the BED is the over-weight, but the psychological problems including feeling guilty, depression and self-hate are very serious too.

But when we are talking about all this eating disorders, we cannot stop thinking about the causes of all these problems. They are many, some of them not explored enough, and we can enumerate social pressure, lack of control, puberty, genetic markers, family influence, emotional distress, depression, low self-esteem and even mass media relentless promotion of a wrong self-image. As the human psyche is very complex, there can be others causes not mentioned here. In every case, there are few causes for an eating disorder, with a dominant one and few secondary one. Let's talk about each category. There are biological factors such as biochemical imbalances and genetic markers, social factors such as cultural and media pressure to one perfect thin image, wrong or limited definition of beauty, discriminatory and stress generating social norms, superficial social norms that elevate good looks over inner qualities and emotional skills. We have interpersonal factors such as long term bullying about appearance or size, difficulties in personal relationships, inability to express feelings, lack of food during childhood, history of physical, sexual or emotional abuse. We have also psychological factors such as anxiety, depression, stress, feeling out of control, feeling inadequate, low self-esteem.

Case study – Zoe

Zoe doesn't have a good opinion about herself, and the self-esteem is almost inexistent. At school she is often teased for being shorter than the rest. All the others are tall, athletic and thin, just like the models from the TV-shows. So Zoe decided to go to the gym, to train herself for hours and adopt a diet low in fat and carbs and high in protein. She is always exhausted, and her mind is thinking obsessively to eat a chocolate bar. Before realizing, the whole bag of chocolate is empty, and she feels disgusted and ashamed, thinking that she endured those long hours of training for nothing. She goes to the toilet and throw up, telling to herself that she will never do it any other time. Starting from tomorrow the diet is on again. It will not take long until this become a vicious circle.

Task: What were the causes for Zoe's eating disorder? Justify your answer.

____

____

____

____

____

So, as we learned, any eating disorder can be caused by one or few more factors described of this chapter. They can interact and create a ripple effect, even if the eating disorder starts due to one factor, let's say genetics, later other factors can be augmented by association. The person suffering from an eating disorder can be emotionally unstable, creating a chemical imbalance with the wrong eating habits, affecting her feelings even more. There is a causal link between risk factors and eating disorders. Let's see the most important ones:

- Age: the most common range for a person to have an eating disorder is between 18 and 20.
- Dieting: the praise that some people get after losing weight can be addictive, and some will think that the more weight they lose, the more praise they will get, especially if we are talking about someone with low self-esteem.
- Emotional problems: are factors which can increase the potential for an eating disorder, even if they are not food related. If you are anxious, depressed or suffering from OCD, you are more likely to develop an eating disorder.
- Family and friends: if some of your relatives or close friends have had or have an eating disorder, chances are that you can develop one too.
- Leisure: if you have a job/work where being slim is important (athletes, models, dancers), the chance to develop an eating disorder increase.
- Gender: 9 out of 10 people with bulimia are female, 1 of 2000 men have had anorexia, compared with 1 of 250 women. BED affects men and women in equal measure (50%/50%).
- Major life events: transitions, changes and important life events bring emotional distress in a person daily schedule. When you are moving in another home, divorce, get abused, change job of suffer due to a crime, you are more likely to develop an eating disorder.

What can we expect when the average runway model is considered to be anorexic by any dietician, with a very low BMI? Under the mass media pressure, promoting a thin, perfect body, most of the people, especially the young women, start to create a wrong body image. This can impact even further in their life, due to the fact that a link exists between what we eat and what we feel, and while this is a natural, normal phenomenon, in the light of an eating disorder, can become distorted and perverted, leading to health issues and death, in some rare cases. One suffering from binge eating disorder could feel depressed, unhappy, uncomfortable or guilty, after a binge that resulted in gaining weight. One full cycle contains a part when they eat excessive amounts of food and a part when they are dieting and even doing exercise to reduce their body fat percentage and weight. In the case of bulimia nervosa, the cycle is a bit different, with the part where some is eating in excess, and the second part called purging, where they vomit or use laxatives to remove the food. They can feel depressed and uncomfortable too. In the case of somebody suffering from anorexia nervosa, the situation is a bit different, there is no cycle, and they can see the food as something bad, evil, because they are afraid of gaining weight. A person with anorexia will see herself as fat and ugly, will be ashamed of how she is looking, and will aim for some unrealistic idea of self-image. They will eat only as much food as they need to keep going on daily basis. An eating disorder will have both physical and psychological effects on the suffering person. The collateral effect will reach even family and friends of an individual suffering from an eating disorder. Let's start with anorexia, as example, where we can have many different symptoms, but the real cause behind all the problems is a distorted self-image. Because of this projected ideal body image, they will often check their weight, they will eat less and count the calorie intake, they will submit themselves to weight loss programs and diets, they will read about weight loss, sometimes they will have only one or two meals per day or they will use laxatives to keep the weight level down. Psychologically speaking, they will have low confidence and low self-esteem, they can be depressed, socially withdrawn and seduced by the idea of loneliness.

Case study – Matilda

Matilda just reached 18 and she is on a diet. It is something normal for a teenager just before the prom's night. She is thinking to lose few pounds and get some stamina. But Matilda's brother Jamie can see that his sister refuse to eat anything unhealthy and try to skip meals when possible. After dinner, she is doing a high-intensity training in her room or she is going out to run a half-marathon. As siblings, they use to be very close, but lately Matilda is busier than ever, and she is not as chattier as before. Jamie can clearly see that most of her clothes are too big for her now, but she is insisting to exercise a lot every day, because she does not want the pounds to get piled up as before. Most of Matilda's internet sessions are now spent on forums and websites about weight loss, and she is hardily talking with her friends.

Task: Can you write here what anorexia's symptoms Matilda had?

____

____

____

____

____

Here is the answer. Check how many symptoms did you identified correctly.

-Skipping meals
-Too much exercise
-Social withdrawal and isolation
-Obsessive check about weight loss info on internet
-Distorted self-image.

Anorexia is easy to spot, but people suffering with bulimia nervosa can still look normal, not being under or over-weight. Many of the symptoms are, in fact, a direct result of purging (forced vomiting of the food), an action used often by people with bulimia nervosa. In this case they can have dental problems, swollen glands, sore throat, in the other case, when they use laxatives instead of purging, all these symptoms do not appear. Psychosomatic and social symptoms, such as isolation and withdrawal, depression and feeling helpless, are also observed in most of the cases.

Case study – Carley
Carly was diagnosed with bulimia one year ago. Even if her friends and family noticed the personality change and her dramatic weight loss, they are thinking that is all due to the school pressure and her being a teenager. Because they care about her, the parents try to lift up her mood by complimenting her about the slim appearance, even if they think that she is exaggerating a bit. Carly is trying hard to not tell anyone about her struggle

with bulimia, as she is thinking that no one will really understand her motives. She is planning her meals accordingly, with a toiler needed to be there close to her eating place, so she is limiting herself to visit other new, interesting, unfamiliar places. She is not smiling anymore, as her teeth decay will make her uncomfortable to do this. Her self-esteem is plummeting down, and the obsession with her self-image and food dealing made her to stop seeing her closest friends lately.

But not only the female side is suffering from this kind of illness. After some increasing pressure to have the perfect body and less body fat, after the professional athlete body image being promoted intensively by mass media, the percentage of male population affected by an eating disorder is growing twice as fast as the female group. Statistically speaking, 19 out of 100.000 males had anorexia nervosa, 29 out of 100.000 males had bulimia nervosa, and 2% from total cases of B.E.D. (binge eating disorder) are males too. Approx. 1-5% of anorexia sufferers are males, but the percentage increase for boys under 16 reported to girls under 16 is close to 50%.

Binge Eating Disorder is one of the illnesses affecting in equal proportion men and women alike. They usually have periods of overeating, without purging, and eating is dominant in their thoughts. Very often they have some fast gain on weight, as over-eating become a habit and it is happening automatically. Because of all these problems, the people suffering from BED will have a negative, distorted body image. Even if they want to lose weight, the compulsion to eat is very strong, and the willpower by itself is not enough to conquer the battle. As they start bingeing, social and psychological signs start to manifest, such as feeling guilty or upset, isolating themselves or withdrawal from the social scene. This can create a vicious circle, as people suffering from BED will eat for comfort when they are upset or guilty. The emotional part of an eating disorder was extensively studied. People suffering from BED feel guilt and disgust after a period of seclusion and excessive eating, but this is not happening because they are uneducated or unable to choose a healthy food, or because of complete lack of self-control. This is a complex and complicate issue on the psychological level. A person suffering from anorexia nervosa will have a distorted, wrong kind of self-image, seeing themselves as ugly and overweight, and they will not like how their body looks. This can lead to depression. The food is something bad and teriffiant, because can make them fat. If one is suffering from bulimia nervosa, they will most often feel guilty and unhappy because of their lifestyle choice especially after bingeing. This can also lead to depression and to them being uncomfortable with their own image. In the same time, one suffering from binge eating disorder can also feel guilty or unhappy after consistently over-eating, leading to weight gain. They will feel depressed and unable to accomplish their goals (goals that are sometimes too high), because of the power of the inner compulsion. And this is not something we can ignore, as The Institute of Child Health and King's College London research will point out that UK number of diagnoses of eating disorders has risen with 15% since 2000, and the percentage of males suffering from an eating disorder has risen by 27%.

Case study - Rose

Rose has an eating disorder. She is 32 and lives alone with her cat Felix. She found her life uneventful, as she moved here four years ago and all her family remained in New Zeeland. She has only a handful of friends, as Rose is working for long hours in a management position. Most of her free time is spent in front of the TV, watching her favorite shows. She is very often too tired to go out, so she isn't expanding the circle of friends. In relation with the food, we are talking about a duality in perceiving the food as both comforting friend and biggest enemy. Rose want to have a healthy approach to her diet, but after she is over-eating, she is feeling guilty and conflicted. She is thinking to find a way to deal with her destructive emotions and to handle the compulsion and the intense feelings of stress and depression.

Task: What eating disorder do you think Rose fight with? What are the reasons for your answer.

____

____

____

____

____

There is another matter to discuss, from a psychological point of view, and that is the effect of a person suffering from an eating disorder on family, friends, colleagues at work and others. Parents are very affected if a child develops an eating disorder, thinking that is their fault and blaming themselves. Siblings can do that too, feeling guilty because they did not observe faster the behavior of their brother or sister. Friends are trying to help at first, with advice and support, but often this will prove ineffective, and they will feel helpful and isolate themselves from their suffering friend. Partners can react in a similar way with a parent, but they will also experience distrust, because it was not shared, blame and guild because they did not picked up the symptoms earlier. Libido can be very low, and this can result in lack of interest and feeling of falling out of love, eventually leading to separation of them two.

Case study – Candice

Candice is concerned about her sister Daniela. She was always shy, but in the past few weeks she has isolated herself from others, no longer joining family meals, choosing to eat downstairs in her room while reading magazines. She is checking her appearance often in the big mirror and she is on the weighting scale at least twice per day. At the beginning Candice was thinking that Daniela has a new boyfriend and she is trying to impress him, but now the evidence is pointing towards an eating disorder. She is feeling useless and guilty for not acting sooner and for not giving a good advice to her sister. They used to be very close, but now she feels her distant and do not want to push her away even further.

Task: Applying what you already learned, what would you advice Candice? How can she approach the matter sensitively? Write few of your ideas.

____
____
____
____
____

It is not very easy to spot someone suffering from an eating disorder, and after that you need to know what kind of advice to give.

The problem is: how we can manage a specific eating disorder? Each of them needs different approaches, and most of the time others can support a friend or relative with his/her recovery. There are also local resources, organisations and treatments available if one is struggling on his path to success. Eating disorders are hard to endure, not only by the one experience it, but also by their friends and relatives. We can only observe the large scale of damage and suffering and we should know that health professionals and dedicated organisations are there to help with prevention and treatment. They will support both people having an eating disorder and their family and friends. Where we can find all these resources? On the internet, we can read on websites with a good reputation such as NHS or BUPA, on the relevant sections, ask on forums and chat rooms, join Facebook groups, call a helpline, contact a voluntary group or charity, ask a professional about his/her opinion.

One of this is called Food First Initiative (www.bapen.org.uk), and was initially developed in Bedfordshire as a necessary approach to understand and manage malnutrition. They define malnutrition as a state of nutrition in which an imbalance, excess or deficiency of energy, minerals, vitamins or other nutrients can cause measurable adverse effects on body form (shape, size or composition) or tissue, function and clinical outcome. They focus more on the so-called under-nutrition, even if malnutrition also includes obesity. They use something named MUST calculator (which can be found on the website address http://www.bapen.org.uk/screening-and-must/must-calculator). Dehydration is another addressed problem, with signs such as dry mouth and lips, thirst, tiredness, dry loose skin, headaches, heavy colored, strong smelling urine. If you are dehydrated, you can tend to experiment ulcers, loss of appetite, confusion, headaches, incontinence, falls, infection, low blood pressure, constipation. The dehydration test is easy, pinch your skin gently on the back of your hand. It should return back to the initial condition rapidly. If your skin is maintaining its pinched shape for a while and drops back slowly, you are dehydrated. The MUST score can be low (0), medium (1), high (2) or very high (3). If it is low, you just need to weight monthly and have a balanced diet, if it is medium you should eat fortified food and have some nourishing snacks or drinks, if it is high, you should also increase your calories intake by 500/1000 daily. If you check on the website you can find the formula for calculating your score, using BMI, weight loss, acute disease impact and some other questions. You will also find lists of 100 calorie boosters and hydration boosters. I found interesting to learn how to estimate height by measuring ulna length and BMI using mid upper arm circumference.

Help for the families involved in something similar:

Always remember that someone suffering with eating disorders will often need support in seeking help, but they will not necessarily want to seek help themselves. In many cases, it is the family and friends of those with eating disorders to turn to these organisations and charities for advice and guidance in the first instance. According to B-EAT (http://www.b-eat.co.uk/), one of the organisations supporting people who suffer from eating disorders, the number of those seeking treatment has increased dramatically over the last 15 years. You can also look for advice on following websites:

- http://www.nhs.uk/Livewell/eatingdisorders/Pages/eating-disorders-explained.aspx

- http://www.rcpsych.ac.uk/healthadvice/problemsdisorders/anorexiaandbulimia.aspx

There are telephone lines for information and support, provided by specialist organisations, being set up to provide guidance on eating disorders over the phone. These organisations and charities are run by well informed, caring and compassionate people, trained in the field of eating disorders, willing to help others. To name a few, everybody heard about B-Eat, Samaritans and Eating Disorders Support.

We need to be careful in searching about this online, as "eating disorders" Key search on Google will generate millions of results. It is important to know where we can find helpful information and where it is just mentioned for traffic gain. NHS website, as well as the websites of different associations and charities, is a good source of information. Some of them got chat-rooms and forums where people suffering from eating disorders, friends and family can talk online and share their experiences. These can be a helpful source of advice and support.

In order to find reliable sources that you can trust, use common sense. Is this one established institution? How old it is the article? What does it shows on their website? Some websites will also contain chat rooms or forums, where people suffering from eating disorders, their family or friends can talk to each other about their experiences. There are also many voluntary groups and charities offering support in UK. B-EAT is a national charity with support groups all around the country. The National Centre for Eating Disorders is an organization which offers counseling, support and advice for carers and friends of people with eating disorders. There are regional organizations too, such as Syeda in South Yorkshire and FEDS Kirklees, just to give some examples.

It is very important that we facilitate the one suffering from eating disorders to meet a professional as soon as possible, in order to start the recovery process. Talking with people possessing the appropriate medical expertise is essential. If you are in need of advice, college or school nurse can help you to do this, staff in walk-in centers and GPs can provide the same service.

Case Study – Kristine

Let's see how professionals helped Kristine with her problem.

She begins crash dieting at age of 16, and she was very self-conscious about her appearances. It was not long before she started to avoid food and missing meals on purpose as often as she could. Her dramatic weight loss could not hide her actions for long, but supported by her father, she visited a nurse, working out her BMI, did some blood tests and was questioned about her severe weight loss. Later on, Kristine was diagnosed with Anorexia and referred to a dietician, a psychiatrist related to Child and Adolescent Mental Health Services (CAMHS). After several sessions, with the specialists help and support, she worked out a diet plan to get her back to a healthy weight. Remember that nurses from school or college, pastoral staff, workers in walk-in center and GPs have the knowledge and expertise to find out the best way to access the right treatment. The patient will need a lot of support and inner strength, struggling to fight against habits grounded deep inside his/her psyche.

Common Strategies to use in recovery:

A. Listen to your family member, colleague or friend. Be inquisitive and insist to discuss, as they may not be ready to share everything yet. It will show that you care about and you support them.
B. Keep the same routines. Do not keep tabs on them at lunch time and try to be there if they need you, but do not make it obvious. Focusing on the illness can slow the recovery. Be positive.
C. Have patience. The process is not always smooth, there are bumps in the road, and they will need your support all the time, knowing that it is someone there to help will greatly improve the odds.
D. Do your research. Find informations and ask others that already went through the recovery. If you find this difficult, ask any organization or charity available in your area. Then you can be at least partially prepared for what is next.

Anorexia

Do not watch a recovering anorexic eating or force them to eat when they do not want to do it. Pressuring them will often have the reverse result. Never compare them with others, as this can reinforce the negative habit, lowering their self-esteem. Most of the people fighting these illnesses feel incapable and inferior, anorexia being a way to gain a measure of control in their own life. Promoting independence and supporting them to have their own plan or strategy is an important step. Praise and encouragement will also result in better coping with the struggle and low self-esteem.

Binge eating disorders (BED)

Help the individual to socialize and take part in group activities in their free time, being in the company on other people will distract them from the nagging thinking about food and encourage to enjoy the company of their friends, more than the simplistic thought that BED is often the result of boredom and loneliness. Creating a routine or implementing a positive habit is very effective when you are dealing with proper eating. Three main meals and healthy snacks in between should be more than enough, but this matter needs all the diplomacy that you can fathom. You do not need to supervise them constantly, sometimes just stocking the cupboard and fridge with nutritious, healthy food – mainly fruits and vegetables – will do the trick. Do not try to make them to diet, as this is a recipe for failure. Food restriction will only intensify the cravings, making a relapse most probable.

Bulimia

Nature heals. Suggest pleasant outdoor activities, to prove that life it is not only about eating. Walking along a river, interval running or hiking a hill or mountain will prove to be a good distraction. As they are often disappearing right after dinner to get rid of the food, encouraging joining small activities after a meal will be a good opportunity to change the usual patterns. Emotional support is as important as the knowledge that they can have a conversation or a game of cards, to stop the constant internal noise and calm the mind. Mindfulness exercises can be helpful too, as long as they are not too long or daunting. Being a role model is good also, eating a nice, balanced meal, allowing yourself a cheat food now and then without feeling guilty can ease the struggle and make them to enjoy eating again.

CHAPTER 6

FOOD SAFETY PRINCIPLES
IN HOME ENVIRONMENT

How to handle the food safely and why is this important? What are the hazards related to food safety? How can we avoid contamination during storage, preparation, cooking, serving or re-heating?

Health problems related to food contamination are increasing in the last 30 years, and they can be as mild as a common nausea or headache, or as dangerous as kidney failure or even death. Researchers in food related healthcare believe that the main reasons for these problems are: changes in shopping pattern, catering for many others, microwaveable and fast cooking pre-packed meals, fast food, preferences for outdoor eating (barbecue), globalization and global scale movement of food ingredients. But, if you learn the basic food safety and hygiene, you should be able to prevent contamination and handle the food in the way that it will make it significantly safe to eat. The reverse is also true, lacking the knowledge will increase the chance of contamination and food related illnesses. The Food Standards Agency reported over one million cases of food related illnesses, resulting in more than 20.000 hospital admissions and over 500 deaths. The estimated cost on the health budget in England and Wales only was 1.6 billion pounds. (More about it on www.cieh.org or on www.nhs.uk websites). There are estimates that more than 1% of UK population suffers from some sort of allergy. There are many causes of food poisoning, and they can group in different categories:

-Allergenic: any food that can cause an allergic reaction, such as nuts, shellfish, strawberries. Allergens can pose a life threatening risk to individuals suffering from food allergies, as they can experience throat swelling, breathing problems and potential collapse (resulting in death from anaphylactic shock). You must always check the labels before cooking for a potential allergic person. Nuts, fish, soy, strawberries and milk are some of the most common causes of allergy. Just to be warned, you need only a small amount of them to cause a severe reaction.

-Chemical: there are some chemicals that can harm if mixed with food, such as sprays and cleaning agents. If we have chemicals used and stored incorrectly and carelessly, there is a risk that sooner or later they may come in contact with food. Just to give one example, an open tin of acidic food like lemon based food can oxidize the metal tin and contaminate whatever it is inside. You can contaminate your food in your own house if you regularly use bleach, cleaning solutions, metal residues or insect repellents in an inadequate way. You can have your food contaminated as a direct result of farming or agriculture (antibiotics used for livestock or pesticides sprayed on crop).

-Bacterial: bacteria can grow as a direct result of faulty hygiene habits, such as not washing your hands before handle food or not storing the food properly, at the right temperature. These changes are difficult to spot, as some of them can be caused by enzymes of micro-organisms (bacteria, viruses, yeasts or molds). There is a type of harmful bacteria named pathogenic bacteria, which may make food inedible or a hazard to health.

-Foreign bodies: they can make their way into mixing with food during manufacturing or they are not removed before consumption (fish bones, animal bones, and small pests).Foreign bodies may include, but not be limited to, pieces of plastic, wood, metal or food packaging contaminating during or after production. Organic items like bones, shells, stalks, pips or stones need to be removed in the preparation process. The lists are quite exhaustive, and let's not forget hair, plasters, jewelry, or pets bringing their hair, droppings or saliva in the mix. Cross contamination can occur when the hazards are spread between people, food, and equipment or work surfaces. The main ways of contamination can happen from person to person, person to food, food to person or food to food.

We should focus on how to minimize the hazardous contaminants to make their way into the food. Even small things like sneezing or holding hands can have a huge impact on food. There are some logical steps that can be taken in order to process and preserve the food safely. We are unable to perceive the harmful bacteria with our senses before they reach a critical mass, we cannot smell it, taste it or see it. So, we need to prepare adequately. The stages or areas of food hygiene and safety are:

- Storage: every food has its own ideal storage conditions. Learn about this or you will store it inappropriately and the food will become fast unusable or inedible.

- Preparation: there are different stages that are linked during food preparation, and contamination can occur at any stage. The bigger impact on the food will be the result of the personal hygiene or the one preparing it.

- Cooking: if the food is not cooked at a high enough temperature, bacteria can survive and multiply, and whoever will eat undercooked food can be poisoned. Cooking it thoroughly can destroy all the harmful bacteria.

- Serving the food: as the person serving the food, you should ensure that the food does not go cold, no one will touch the food they do not intend to eat and perishable meals are not left at room temperature for more than 2 hours.

- Reheating: if you are constantly reheating the food, as tempting as it may be, the harmful bacteria will multiply. Only reheat food twice, at a minimum of 75 degrees Celsius (82 in Scotland). Use a food thermometer to check it.

Maintaining personal hygiene, when you handle food, will ensure the safety of the cook and the ones eating the food. You can carry bacteria both inside and outside the human body, so your standards should be very high. Cleaning hands is of paramount importance, as one effective technique to be used. Hair can contaminate food physically, so you need to use nets, hats or other forms of head covering to prevent it. You should ensure that your nails are clean and short, no fake nails or nail varnish, as they can drop off in the food. A big percentage of population is a passive carrier of Staphylococcus Aureus, in our nose, mouth or ears. We should avoid coughing or sneezing around food, picking nose, using a spoon multiple times to tasted or using our fingers, smoking during our cooking session or having open cuts, boils or spots. In most of the places you need to use specialist protective clothing, such as hairnets, overalls or aprons, gloves, anti-slip shoes. At home, you should take the adequate measures and dress properly before starting to cook. Jewelry like rings, bracelets, watches, all of them can contaminate food through the bacteria and dirt or by dropping physical bits of jewelry in the food. It is better if you remove anything that it is not necessary when cooking. If you contaminate your hands, the bacteria will spread quickly around the kitchen. Always use warm water and antibacterial soap when washing hands. There is a correct way to wash your hands, and you can search about it online. You are required to wash your hands before starting to cook, before handling food, between touching raw and ready-made food, after handling raw food, after handling waste, after going to toilet, after touching chemicals or money, after taking lunch or going for break, after eating, coughing, sneezing or smoking. This will significantly increase the food safety.

Case study – Juliet

Being Sunday, Juliet is waking up feeling good, as the week is coming to an end, and she will be in holiday from Monday. She wake up at 6, but she will start work at 8.30. As it is early, she will wash her hands and cook some pasta for lunch pack, while eating a Marmite sandwich. Once done, she washed her hands once more and leaves for the bus. First thing when arriving, Juliet goes to the toilet, and then she washes her hands and starts to cook. Later in the afternoon, the team manager asks her if she can thoroughly clean the kitchen, as it is on the day schedule. She will collect all the rubbish and take it to the bin, wiping all the surfaces and checking the fridge and freezer temperature. She will wash one more time before going to the staff room to collect her jacket and bag.

Once at home, she will cook a nice family dinner, making hunters chicken, and washing the hands before and after handling the meat. Once dinner is prepared, she will change her clothes and get everything ready. His newborn nephew is coming to visit with his parents, so she is not taking any chances related to the food hygiene.

Not caring about those elementary rules, there is a high change that food will be contaminated. Even if we talk about a foreign object such as bone or piece of glass, they can physically harm the person eating the food.

Which are the most common bacteria, what are the symptoms and the onset time and how can we avoid it?

A. Bacillus Cereus, found in cereals, pasta and rice, or if you accidentally ingest dust or soil. Can induce vomiting, diarrhea and stomach pain. The onset time is 1-5 hours in case of food, 8-22 hours for dust and soil. Can be avoided by proper cooking and cooling down the food, or by not storing rice at room temperature for long periods of time.

B. Clostridium botulinum can be found in fish, meat, veggies, peanut butter and soil. Ingested, can lead to diarrhea, stomach ache, eyesight problems, impaired swallowing and breathing, paralysis and, in rare cases, death. The onset time is 12-36 hours, and you can avoid this washing everything thoroughly and by not using damaged cans. You need also to cook and preserve food properly.

C. Clostridium perfringens can found in raw meat, animal waste, insects remains, soil and dust. Can induce stomach aches and diarrhea. The onset time is 8-18 hours. You can avoid by keeping raw and cooked foods separated, clean thoroughly and cook and cool down the food carefully.

D. Salmonella can be found in raw meat, especially poultry, eggs, unpasteurized milk, animal guts, rodents and sewage. Can induce fever, vomiting, diarrhea and stomach ache. Onset time is 13-36 hours. In order to avoid it, you need to keep the raw and cooked food separated, maintain a general cleanliness, store food at safe temperature and keep the pets away from the food.

E. Staphylococcus Aureus can be found in human nose and mouth, untreated milk. Can induce severe vomiting, diarrhea, stomach ache. Onset time is 1-7 hours. To avoid it, you need to wash hands before after you touch yours or somebody else's face, avoid coughing or sneezing around food, cover you cuts.

F. Campilobacter Jejuni can be found in raw meat, chicken, animals and birds, untreated milk or water. Can induce diarrhea, stomach aches, headache and nausea. Onset time is 2-5 days. Can be avoid if you cook your food at the right temperature, separate the raw and cooked food, maintain cleanliness and pasteurize the milk.

G. Shigellosis (dysentery) is found in water of food contaminated with human feces. Can induce diarrhea (blood is present in some cases), stomach aches. Onset time is 1-7 days. You avoid it by cleaning toilets thoroughly, not sharing hand towels, washing fruit and veg properly in clean water.

H. E Coli is found in raw or undercooked meat, untreated dairy products and after contact with farm animals. They can give you diarrhea, stomach aches and sometimes severe kidney problems. Onset time is 3-4 days. Can be avoided by keeping the raw and cooked food separated and cooking the food at the right temperature, especially burgers and sausages.

I. Listeria can be found in unpasteurized dairy, meat pate, soil and contaminated water. Can induce fever, diarrhea, stomach aches, and, in rare cases, blood poisoning and meningitis. If you are pregnant can cause a miscarriage. The onset time is 3-70 days. Warning: Pregnant women should avoid the meals carrying listeria risk. Check use by dates. Store at the right temperature.

J. Norovirus is highly infectious, airborne and can contaminate water. Manifest as fever, diarrhea, and stomach pains. Onset time is 12-48 hours, can be avoided through proper cleaning of toilets and not sharing hand towels, and by maintaining a proper cleanliness of the place.

How are we storing the food safely? To begin with, we need to categorize the food as fresh, convenience, low risk and high risk. When we bring the food into our home, we should check for hazards, use only suppliers with excellent reputation, the food needs to be labeled and not contaminated by anything. Then you need to proceed with correct storage in your home. What you can do? Refrigeration, as refrigerating is one of the most common storage methods. What you need to know about? High risk, perishable foods should be always refrigerated, to avoid bacteria to multiply faster. Hot food should be cooled down first, as condensation can contaminate the other containers with food. Raw meat, poultry and fish should be stored on bottom of the fridge. Next is the ready-to-eat food, which needs to be stored separately than the raw ones. Fresh salad and vegetables should be stored in boxes with lid, to avoid contamination from raw food drips. Just for a fact, after WWII, only 2-3% of the UK homes owned a fridge, by 2015, the number went up to almost 100%.

I mentioned high risk and low risk food. The high risk one is usually the cooked, ready to eat – food. This kind of food is an ideal environment for the bacteria development, and if it is contaminated, the numbers of harmful bacteria will grow exponentially. As we are often not cooking it again, we should keep those foods at low temperature, and only for a short period outside the fridge. This category include cooked prawns or crabs, sushi, meat or kidney pie, cream or milk cakes, cold ham, pasta, rice pudding and other similar meals. The low risk ones do not support the bacteria growth and they are not causing food poisoning in normal circumstances. As opposed to **use by date** for high risk food, they will have a **best before date.** They can be stored in cool, clean, dry areas, away from sunlight, and not necessarily in the fridge. Chocolate, sweets, crisps, cans, tins and sauce like ketchup or barbecue are the ones in this low risk category.

Pre-packed food – have a date marking when is safe and in the best condition to be used. As I specified before, the date marks can be divided in two categories. Use by – for perishable food, and eating it after this date can put you at risk. It is an offence to sell food past the use by date. The second category is Best Before, and it is merely showing a date within which the food is expected to be optimal. You can find this one especially on items like biscuits and crisps. You can also find on the label informations about how to store the items. The date mark is useful only if the food is stored correctly. We can have different demands: sweets can be stored in a cool, dark place, mayonnaise needs to be kept in the fridge and ice cream cakes need to be put in the freezer at -22 degrees. This is one of the ways to reduce the risk of food poisoning or spoiling the food and safekeeping the taste and the structural integrity.

Task: Collect the labels of five different foods and check the expiring date and how they need to be stored.

____

____

____

____

____

The next step on our journey is the nutritional value and how this will change in relationship with how it is stored. So, it is also important to store them properly, not only to avoid food poisoning, but to ensure that the nutrients are not destroyed in the process. If you want to find more, you need to search about "retention factors" – the numbers showing how the food retains or loses its nutrients. One of the places to start to learn about it is the USDA (United States Department of Agriculture) website.

Light exposure is one of the factors that can affect the nutritional value of the food, leading to a significant decrease of nutrients like vitamins, proteins, fats and pigments. A sure way to avoid this is to store the food in a dark place. Temperature is another one, and while a lower temperature will deteriorate the nutrients from fruits or milk, a higher one can make bacteria to thrive and multiply exponentially, resulting in chemical reactions that destroy some vitamins or break down protein, or just cause food poisoning due to the higher number count. Oxygen is also a cause of food spoilage and nutrients deterioration, with adverse effects on flavour, vitamins and fats. It is always better to keep food in airtight containers or nicely wrapped, to avoid bacteria growth and enzymatic reactions that spoil the food. Water can be a good support for bacteria development, so some foods are dehydrated of frozen to keep them for longer periods, This is one of the reasons behind the requirement to store food in dry places, and following the label instructions will make you to avoid further deterioration of a specific food. Imagine that, due to the incorrect storage, more than 7 million tons of food is thrown away every year in UK only. Freezing is another option to minimize nutrients loss, which sometimes works better than other methods. Just to compare, vitamin A lose 5% by freezing, 50% by drying, 25% after cooking, 36% if you cook and drain and 10% more every time you reheat. Iron, by comparison, will lose only 35% when cooking and 40% if you cook and drain. If you are an athlete, pregnant, diabetic, and vegetarian or vegan, you should learn more about the retention measurement.

Next step into avoid food poisoning is to keep the kitchen clean and to dispose of food waste efficiently. The purpose of a hygienic and properly cleaned food work area is to prevent the food contamination. The cross contamination occurs when bacteria travel from one food to another, or from hands, equipment or surfaces. The multiplying bacteria can pose a threat to your health. In one of his experiments, a scientist called C. Gerba found out that sponges, dish cloths and chopping boards contains on average more bacteria than a toilet seat. As an example of cross contamination, we can have some raw meat touching or dripping into another food, equipment, work surface and cook's clothes, then ready to eat meal come in contact with something dripped by raw meat.

Task: Next time when you prepare a meal in your kitchen, for the whole preparation process, make a list of the food work areas or other items that can become contaminated or cross contaminate after the process is finished.

The aim of a clean and hygienic food work area is to prevent food contamination, to eliminate the conditions that cause the bacterial growth, to minimize the possibility of cross contamination, to reduce the bacteria to a safe level and to avoid the environment to become attractive to pests and vermin. An efficient approach to this could be done, by cleaning up as soon as the food preparation is done, by cleaning and disinfecting the equipment after every use, by cleaning every area that is in no direct contact with food according to a schedule (think bins and floor). Items like fridge, freezer and the area inside and around them should be done ideally every week. A good cleaning schedule will imply what you need to clean, how often, what is the best way to do it, when to disinfect, how often and in which way, and do not forget to think at what items to use for cleaning and disinfection. We need detergents to break down fats and dirt, but they do not kill bacteria, disinfectants to kill bacteria, but they do not break down the fats and dirt, and sanitizers to reduce the number of bacteria. The food should be put away before cleaning with chemical cleaners, we should wear protective clothing if required, never to mix chemicals, store them separately, clearly labeled and out of children reach. Other helpful method to minimize cross contamination is to use color coded chopping boards, one color being assigned exclusively for one type of food. You can disinfect using hot water or steam at temperature over 80 degrees, or chemical disinfectants, as per instructions provided (contact time with the surface, rinse time, wipe time). The areas with a high risk of cross contamination such as food contact surface, equipment or fixture that may be touched by food and hands should be the main focus of our disinfection process. Special care to equipment used to clean the food work area such as clothes, mops, bins, as they will be in contact with contaminants and must not transfer them elsewhere.

Here are few pointers related on how to maintain your kitchen safe:

Worktops – always wash them before starting to prepare food, wipe up any food spillage right away, always wash properly after you use it for raw eggs, poultry or other meat and avoid to put salad, bread or fruits on a worktop that you used for raw meat. You can use a dishwasher to clean a chopping board effectively. It is ideal to use separate ones for raw meat and for other types of food.

Clothes for cleaning – you should try to have separate clothes for any jobs, one for chopping board, one for dishes and so on. Or you can use disposable kitchen towel, so it is less likely for bacteria to spread on other items or clothes. It is very important to wash and change them regularly, and dry them well. Tea towels and sponges can also spread bacteria, so the previous rule applies to them too. It is very easy to touch raw meat, clean with a towel and use it later for another dish, spreading the bacteria.

Kitchen utensils – you can understand why it is important to wash them thoroughly after every use, especially after raw meat. If you have a dishwasher the problem is solved, if not wash them with hot water and disinfectant/washing up liquid.

Hands – are the easiest way to contaminate the food because we are touching so many things when we are cooking (food, fridge handle, towels, can opener and many others). You should always wash the hands after going to toilet, after touching the bin or touching pets, after touching raw food such as meat, vegetables or eggs and of course, before starting to cook. Dry them properly, ideally with disposable kitchen towels, and definitely don't use your apron for it.

Cooking food at the right temperature

On every recipe you can find the time and temperature needed for a meal to be prepared, but those are only general guidelines and should not be presumed to be right for similar types of food. Doesn't matter if you prefer your food hot or cold, you should always cook it at the right temperature. This way it will be safe and bacteria free. Just to give you an example, one single bacteria can become a colony of 15.000.000 in half a day. When we are referring at this number of harmful bacteria, you can get critically, life threatening ill. Warming a food up to 55-60 degrees Celsius will multiply the bacteria, instead of killing it, making that meal a fertile breeding ground for bacteria. To be out of the danger zone, the food core needs to be warmed up to more than 75 degrees Celsius. You can use a food thermometer to check your cooking, and if you need to reheat, only reheat it once. If you use the microwave, you should stir at the half-time, in order to make sure that your meal is evenly cooked. If the food was contaminated during the preparation, we should use the right temperature to kill all the bacteria. If you use a probe thermometer, do not forget to clean it and disinfect it after usage. Steaming it or placing it in boiling water will ensure that the probe is clean. You can also check the accuracy this way. The thermometer should display 100 degrees Celsius in boiling water. If you place it in ice, it should display 0(zero) degrees Celsius. One degree in plus or minus is acceptable, more than that means that our probe is inaccurate. Never use a mercury thermometer for food, as you can contaminate it with heavy metals.

Now, let's talk about food waste. This is one of the main first world problems, and until we learn how to dispose of food properly, it will be costly and wasteful on a social scale. According to WRAP (The Waste and Resources Action Programme), UK private households dispose of 7 million tons of food every year, and this is the equivalent of 20% of all the food that it is purchased. Approximately 4 million tons of this food could have been used (and this is the equivalent of 13 billion portions). What is the next step? Reduce the amount of food that you buy, less in bulk and more often. Learn how to dispose of food in a clean, safe and hygienic mode, in order to prevent cross contamination, as the unwanted food can be easily become a place where bacteria is thriving, and food pests such as mice, rats, flies, cockroaches and ants can spread the contamination even further. Rinse out food containers and tins in order to minimize decomposition and bacteria growth. Remove air as much as possible when you wrap, as lack of oxygen will delay the bacterial growth and reduce the unpleasant odors. Food waste needs to be double wrapped before being placed into the bin, to avoid attracting pests. Use black bin bags to easily remove and transport the waste. Empty regularly, have a food pedal if possible and clean it and disinfect it often. Do not keep the bin close to your food, close to door or windows and do not use your hands to open and close the lid. Clean the area where the bin is kept, as sometimes waste can spill into the floor. The lid should be well fitted and secured.

For an outside bin, consider usage of bin powders for bacteria and odors, insecticide for flies, and clean it regularly. It is ideal to have a lining at the bottom of the bin, and to keep it in a cool, shadowed place. Have a well fitted lid and close it always.

ABOUT THE AUTHOR

Got my first company at 16, more than 20 years ago. Just a market stall, but still paid all my university expenses. Accountant for 10 years, then, one day i felt enough is enough, and i left everything. Changed countries, start working in healthcare, 6 years from now, advanced from NVQ 1 to 5. Meanwhile i studied yoga for more than 20 years, learn few languages, studied finances and economy trends, become an angel investor on small scale, start to learn about start-ups, shares, bonds, real estate and other boring stuff. Aiming for Tim Ferris four hour workweek, but I'm not quite there. Training towards a life coach, therapist and motivational speaker career. And all that when I'm still travelling around the world, going to any seminar or movie I'm interested to see, being in a meaningful relation and doing exercises few times a week. In my peak state i am an unstoppable genius, at my lowest I'm just a lazy guy who like to watch Game of Thrones or play League of Legends/Heroes of the Storm/Hearthstone. Average person with amazing skills in a crisis situation. Have driving license, but do not like to drive. Anything except maybe an ATV. Still need to learn Chinese, jump with parachute and play an instrument.